week

REFORMING HEALTH CARE SYSTEMS

The Section F Series
British Association for the Advancement of Science

Reforming Health Care Systems

Experiments with the NHS

Proceedings of Section F (Economics) of the
British Association for the Advancement of Science
Loughborough 1994

Edited by

A.J. Culyer

Professor of Economics, University of York, UK

and

Adam Wagstaff

Reader in Economics, University of Sussex, UK

Edward Elgar
Cheltenham, UK • Brookfield, US

© The British Association for the Advancement of Science 1996

Published by
Edward Elgar Publishing Limited
8 Lansdown Place
Cheltenham
Glos GL50 2HU

Edward Elgar Publishing Company
Old Post Road
Brookfield
Vermont 05036
US

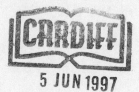

British Library Cataloguing in Publication Data
Reforming health care systems : experiments with the NHS. –
    (The section F series, British Association for the
    Advancement of Science)
    1.National Health Service (Great Britain) – Economic
    aspects   2.Health services administration – Great Britain
    3.Health care reform – Great Britain
    I.Culyer, A.J. (Anthony John), 1942–   II.Wagstaff, Adam
    III.British Association for the Advancement of Science.
    Section F (Economics)
    351.8'41'0941

Library of Congress Cataloguing in Publication Data
Reforming health care systems : experiments with the NHS : proceedings
    of Section F (Economics) of the British Association for the
    Advancement of Science, Loughborough, 1994 / edited by A.J. Culyer
    and Adam Wagstaff.
        p.   cm.— (The Section F series)
    Proceedings of the 1994 meeting.
    Includes index.
        1. Medical care—Great Britain—Finance—Congresses.   2. National
    Health Service (Great Britain)—Economic aspects—Congresses.
    3. Health care reform—Great Britain—Congresses.   I. Culyer, A.J.
    (Anthony J.)   II. Wagstaff, Adam.   III. British Association for the
    Advancement of Science. Section F (Economics)   IV. Series.
    RA410.55.G7R44   1996
    338.4'33621'0941—dc20   95–42419
                                                                                                              CIP

ISBN 1 85898 329 0

Typeset by Manton Typesetters, 5–7 Eastfield Road, Louth, Lincolnshire LN11 7AJ, UK.

Printed and bound in Great Britain by
Hartnolls Limited, Bodmin, Cornwall

Contents

Figures

Tables

Notes on the contributors

Martin Chalkley is a lecturer in economics at the University of Southampton. His current research is concerned with the role of information in the economy, especially with how imperfect information can lead to market failure. He is currently Managing Editor of the *Economic Review*. He enjoys cycling, music and squash – not necessarily in that order.

A.J. Culyer is Head of the Department of Economics and Related Studies, University of York, and Deputy Vice-Chancellor. Status-only Professor, University of Toronto. Member of Central Research and Development Committee of the National Health Service, and of North Yorkshire Health Authority. President (1994) of the Economics Section of the British Academy. Member of Northern and Yorkshire Regional Research Committee. Chair of the Task Force on Supporting Research and Development in the National Health Service (1993–94). Co-editor, *Journal of Health Economics*, on the editorial boards of four other journals and on the editorial board of the Office of Health Economics. He has published 150 articles, 24 books, and 24 pamphlets on health economics and related topics. He spends his spare time as organist and choir trainer in an Anglican parish church.

Cam Donaldson is Deputy Director of the Health Economics Research Unit at the University of Aberdeen. Previously he has held posts at the Centre for Health Economics at the University of York, the Health Care Research Unit at the University of Newcastle upon Tyne and the Department of Public Health at the University of Sydney. His research interests include willingness to pay for health care, financing and organization of health care, the development and application of methods of economic evaluation and using economics in health care priority setting. Cam has acted as a health economics consultant to several local and national NHS bodies as well as to the Medical Research Council. He is also the organizer of the Health Economists' Study Group. Cam is a keen squash player and reluctantly admits to being a season ticket holder at Aberdeen Football Club!

Robert G. Evans is Professor (Economics) at the University of British Columbia; National Health Scientist; Fellow and Director, Program in Population Health; Canadian Institute for Advanced Research. Member, Prime Minister's National Forum on Health, 1994–98; Commissioner, British Columbia Royal Commission on Health Care and Costs, 1990–91. His published books are *Why Are Some People Healthy and Others Not?* New York:

Aldine–de Gruyter, 1994 (edited, with M.L. Barer and T.R. Marmor); and *Strained Mercy: the Economics of Canadian Health Care*, Toronto: Butterworths, 1984.

Jeremy Hurst is a senior economic advisor in the National Health Service Executive. He studied economics at the London School of Economics in the 1960s and specialized in health economics in the early 1970s. In 1981 he spent a year in North America studying alternative ways of financing health care. In 1990 he spent a year at the OECD studying health care reforms, which led to the publication in 1982 of *The Reform of Health Care: A Comparative Analysis of Seven OECD Countries*. His favourite pastimes are travelling and long-distance walking.

Julian Le Grand is the Richard Titmuss Professor of Health Policy at the London School of Economics and Professorial Fellow at the King's Fund Policy Institute. He was previously Professor of Public Policy at the University of Bristol and a lecturer in economics at the London School of Economics and at the University of Sussex. He is the author of many articles and books on the welfare state, including most recently *Quasi-Markets and Social Policy* (with Will Bartlett), Macmillan, 1993, and *Evaluating the NHS Reforms* (with Ray Robinson), King's Fund, 1994.

Alistair McGuire is a reader in economics at City University, London, and a research associate at the Centre for Socio-Legal Studies, Wolfson College, Oxford. He has been intrigued by the complexities of resource allocation within the health care sector for some considerable time. He has published widely in this area and feels he is beginning to have some understanding of the appropriate questions.

James M. Malcomson is Professor of Economics at the University of Southampton. His current research is concerned with contracts and incentives, especially their implications for labour markets (wages, unemployment and trade unions) and for provision of health services. He has published extensively in international journals on these issues. Other activities involve mountains, music and photographs.

David Mayston is Professor of Public Sector Economics, Finance and Accountancy at the University of York, and Director of the new Centre for Performance Evaluation and Resource Management (CPERM) at York. He has previously taught at the Universities of British Columbia, Western Ontario, Essex and Western Australia. He is particularly interested in issues of resource management in health care and education, including capital and labour resources, and issues that straddle management, finance, accounting and economics.

Adam Wagstaff is a reader in economics in the School of Social Sciences at the University of Sussex. He has acted as a consultant to various international organizations, including the OECD, the UNDP, the World Bank and the WHO, and is an associate editor of the *Journal of Health Economics*. His research interests include equity in the finance and delivery of health care, the demand for health and health care, and efficiency measurement.

Foreword

A.J. Culyer and Adam Wagstaff

The 1994 meeting of the British Association for the Advancement of Science
at Loughborough University of Technology afforded the Economics Section
an opportunity to bring to a wider audience some of the current thinking
amongst economists about the great issues involved in the development and
recent reforms of the National Health Service and, indeed, those arising in
health care systems worldwide. These issues comprise, among others, questions of the finance of medical care (who should pay, for what, and through
what types of insurance in combination with what out-of-pocket contributions from users); the effectiveness of medical care (what works, for whom,
under what circumstances, and with what associated costs and risks); the
need for rationing resources (both to professionals like doctors and managers
and to customers like patients and their families); and the wider (or deeper)
determinants of health (that may go well beyond medical care into genetics,
the environment, equality in society and strategies for coping with stress).
This book is the fruit of that opportunity and consists of the written versions
of the lectures given during the conference.

We are extremely grateful to several individuals and organizations for
making the whole thing possible: to the local secretariat, especially Lawrence
Leger, the local Section Secretary, of the Economics Department at Loughborough University of Technology; to the Economics Section Recorder, Douglas Mair of Heriot-Watt Business School; to the Economics Section Committee and its chair Tad Rybczynski of City University; and to the Office of
Health Economics and its Director, Adrian Towse, for its generous sponsor-
ship of the 1994 proceedings. Without each of these, the occasion would not
have been the pleasure and success that it was – and this book would not have
seen the light of day.

We are also extremely grateful to the authors, who not only kept with
astounding self-discipline to the brief given them by the 1994 President
(Culyer) but also adhered to the various deadlines that were set as the project
progressed.

To the reader we would say this: we conjecture that this book will contain a
good many surprises, both about the issues that economists have been addressing (not usually, it must be emphasized, in isolation from others) and the
ways in which they have been approaching them (for example, the economists' discussions of issues of fairness, and their application of ideas of

efficiency are far more comprehensive than is popularly thought to be typical of the 'economic' approach, as is the extent to which they draw on the insights of specialists coming from many different disciplinary and professional backgrounds). We do not aim, of course, merely to surprise, and whether we surprise or not is not a test of the usefulness of the book. We aim also to engage a wider public in the issues with which policy makers at the top of the NHS and in health authorities, as well as operational managers and professionals, have constantly to wrestle; to deepen understanding about the real nature of the problems; to appreciate why there are no easy solutions; and to come to grips with the kinds of choices and trade-offs that are likely to have to be made.

The title adopted for the Section's sessions in 1994 was 'Challenges facing the NHS'. The NHS's challenges are, however, not unique, as the reader who perseveres only a little way into the chapters that follow will discover. What makes the current period so extremely interesting is the variety of responses to these challenges that is found around the world. Everywhere there is change and 'reform'. Everywhere there is concern over cost and 'effectiveness'. Everywhere there is concern about fairness in the distribution and availability of health care to those it serves. But while the general character of the problems is broadly the same everywhere, that cannot be said of the various responses. As a result there is much that the UK has to learn from other countries, just as there is doubtless much that we in the UK have to teach. One common starting point for all that follows is that we do not assume, uncritically, that the NHS is 'the best in the world' or that it has exhausted its capacity for improvement. However, we doubt that simple slogan-mongering, or sentimental attachment to a largely successful history of medicine in the UK, are useful ways forward. One needs to step outside traditional moulds of thought and traditional politics to examine some fundamental beliefs which impede even those who share a common ideal vision of what medicine should be and how it should be delivered, and who share a common commitment to the egalitarianism that has sustained the NHS since its inception after the Second World War. These common values also need examination, not in order to hasten the advent of a new philistinism, but to inject greater clarity into the values that ought to underpin medical and health care practices and delivery systems. Again, simple (even appealing) slogans will not do unless they afford a basis for actual decision-making in and about our health care systems.

If the authors slaughter a few sacred cows as they go along, that is not to be counted a necessarily bad thing: the health of populations is too important a matter to be obstructed by ruminative slow-moving (or sedentary) traffic.

1 The NHS reforms – a challenge or a threat to NHS values?

A.J. Culyer

Introduction

In 1994, the Economics Section of the British Association for the Advancement of Science explored an area that occupies the centre stage of public policy debate. It is also an area where two broad fields of scientific endeavour come together: medicine and economics. As sciences, they have more in common than you may think. Each, for example, asks the usual scientific questions like 'why do we observe particular phenomena and not others?' and 'what can be predicted to happen if ...?'. They also have in common the difficulty of applying strictly controlled experimental methods. There are important examples of empirical testing and analysis in both subjects, but there are also huge areas where it has not been used (with the consequence that much that is done in medicine does not have substantive empirical backing) and many areas where it is extremely difficult to use (for example, assessing the consequences of the NHS reforms for economic efficiency is too complicated a task to be in any comprehensive sense a researchable topic). The two sciences also have in common the interrelatedness of non-scientific and scientific questions. The sort of non-scientific question I have in mind is that which uses the word 'ought'. Ought the NHS to extend screening programmes for preventable diseases? Ought the NHS to charge patients for home visits by GPs? Because of this intertwining of what is sometimes called the positive (that is, the scientific) with the normative (that is, the ethical), we must all be clear about the nature of the discourse that we are having at any particular moment. Scientists, whether medical or economic, are not necessarily the best people to answer ethical questions (and it is all too easy for a spurious scientific authority to be given to what may be pretty arbitrary and personal value-judgements). Moreover, the attention that is given to ethical questions, particularly so that they may be given answers that can be acceptably embodied in policy, is often scant. As a result, confusion reigns supreme in crucial areas.

Life in the NHS has rarely been unexciting or unchallenging. It has reached fever-pitch in the last fifteen years. Since the publication of *Working for Patients* in 1989 (the White Paper that set the scene for the great changes that have ensued since then) there have been massive changes in the objectives set for the NHS, the ways in which they are to be met, in organization and management, and in the mode of financing health care in the UK. At present we are going through a further set of changes that will leave scarcely anything familiar untouched: funding is again to be changed; management, especially at regional level, is undergoing restructuring; private services are likely to be increasingly commissioned by the NHS; R&D is to be reorganized. Even at the level with which everyone is familiar – the general practitioner – radical changes are taking place. The UK is not unique in experiencing massive change – nor in experiencing change upon change. Neither is it unique in that it is responding to pressures on costs that arise from public expectations and advancing medical technology. Similar pressures exist elsewhere in both the developed and less developed world. Yet the NHS is, of course, unique in the details of its changes. Our experiments, if that is the right word to describe them, are ours alone and many of the paths we are following are uniquely ours, flowing partly out of our own history, partly out of our values, and partly out of the special vision that Conservative governments have more or less consistently brought to bear on health policy – or, more specifically, health care policy.

Gaps in understanding

Despite these massive changes, I detect huge gaps in understanding. These gaps are all-pervading; they exist not only between what the government is seeking to achieve and its comprehension by the general public, but also between the government and the professionals who work in the NHS, among those professional groups that support the service through medical, nursing, and other forms of training activity and between those at, so to speak, the coal face and the research community. Moreover, there are not just gaps in understanding; there are also outright myths. One of them is that, since the NHS was established after the Second World War, there has been greater equality of health in the UK. That is not at all the case, as we have known since the Black Report of 1980 (Department of Health and Social Security 1980) and from other studies (e.g. Marmot et al. 1991). Indeed, gaps in life expectancy and health between social classes, and even between more specific gradings of people (for example, civil service grades), have been *widening*, not narrowing. I shall have something to say about these inequalities later.

I shall not attempt to account for the gaps in understanding, though I have little doubt that there is no single reason for them. But let me try at least to illustrate some of them. Take the gap between what the government is trying to do and the public perception of it. The latter is at best muddled. The key fact is that since the beginning of this decade a crucial split has been created between those in the NHS who commission health care on behalf of us all (the health authorities and the fundholding GPs) and those, whether in the public or private sector, who provide the patient services, whether preventive or curative, hospital- or community-based. The three main ideas behind this split are simple. First, under the old system, the professional providers had 'captured' the system. It had become largely driven by professional priorities and interests rather than those of the people for whom the NHS exists: its patients, current and potential. Second, there was no clear point in the old system at which the community's needs for health care were identified and articulated. This is now clearly the job of the purchasing health authorities (and GPs) and it is their priorities rather than those of the professionals that increasingly dominate. The mechanism is the classic one: *purchasers have the money*. Hospitals and community services are funded only to the extent that the purchasing authorities see a need for them. To my mind, this was the most fundamental element of the reforms. For the first time a service dedicated to the equitable meeting of the community's needs for health care now has a powerful organizational tier with the task of doing just that. The third idea is to encourage competition between providers for the custom of the health authorities and the GPs, and more or less formal agreements, loosely termed contracts, between them which specify as best they can the types and amounts of service to be provided, their location, their quality, and their cost. The objective here is to increase both volume and quality without increasing cost in proportion. In principle – and increasingly in practice – the service providers who win these contracts can be private sector providers, either for profit or not.

My experience, in talking informally to people from ordinary walks of life, is that there is a woeful ignorance about this split and its hoped-for consequences. Many seem to believe that health services have somehow become 'commercialized', with cheapness and profit becoming the touchstones of success and the tradition of free services at the point of need in imminent danger of being swept away. But you don't have to be a slavish government supporter to see that this is wholly false: the intention is to squeeze out ineffectiveness and inefficiency, to target resources where they are most needed, and to use a quasi-market mechanism as just one of several mechanisms to achieve these aims. There is no logical implication whatsoever that patient charges should follow, nor that private insurance for health care follows, nor that private provision is inherently better than public. It is true that the changes in general practice have begun to produce what seems to be a two-tier service that favours NHS patients registered with fundholding GPs. But, serious though this is, it is not of the essence of the reforms; nor is it an objective of them. It is partly a problem of transition, as the number of fundholders rises relative to the number of old-style GPs, and it is partly an ongoing problem (unless and until every GP becomes a fundholder or a member of a consortium of fundholders) which ought to be substantially resolved once the Family Health Service Authorities (which fund the GPs) are merged with the health authorities.

Is the NHS efficient?
I have just mentioned ineffectiveness and inefficiency – the language of economists, accountants and other men (mostly they are men) in grey suits. But surely the NHS is one of the most efficient health care systems in the world? Don't we spend much less on health care than most other countries of similar wealth and suffer no apparent relative harm to our health as a result? The NHS *is* one of the most efficient systems in the world today. We spend less per head than many other countries do. Moreover, we do not suffer the US nightmare in which the spending per head is huge (nearly three times ours) while about 30 per cent of the people are excluded from the right to care (and are dependent on charity). But these facts do not imply that the NHS is as efficient or effective as it could be. All systems, everywhere, are fairly inefficient at the fundamental job of maximizing the impact of health care resources (whatever their size) on the people's health. Nor does it follow that, just because we spend less per head than any developed country apart from Ireland, Spain and Portugal, we spend that money well. It is another myth that merely pumping more resources into health care, willy-nilly, without regard to the effectiveness of what it will accomplish in terms of people's health, is what is needed to improve the nation's health in general. It is also a myth that the reforms are preventing the extra spending that many nonetheless feel is needed. It is much more plausible to suppose the reverse: as and when the reforms focus resources where they do most good – that is, effectively meeting needs – then (and only then) does the case for a higher rate of real growth in health spending begin to become convincing.

It is also a myth that the advent of the NHS itself ushered in a period beginning in the 1940s in which health inequalities in the UK have diminished. The health differences between people of different social status are widening. People in the lowest socioeconomic group have about 10 per cent less life than those in the top group. In 1931 the top group (professional people) had a standardized (age-adjusted) mortality rate (SMR) of 90 per cent of the average, while the lowest group (unskilled) had an SMR of 111 per cent. By 1981 the top rate had fallen to 66 per cent and the bottom rate had risen to 166 per cent. Even amongst civil servants, none of whom could be considered seriously deprived, there is a persisting inverse relationship between grade and health – both length and quality of life (for a discussion see Wilkinson 1986). This trend is not one that was introduced by Conservative governments. It seems to have been under way since the 1930s.

Ethical issues

I now turn to another and quite different sort of problem that lies at the heart of our difficulties in closing the gap in understanding. This time it's a philosophical problem, but not an ivory-tower problem. Failure to resolve this problem will probably lead to the biggest myth-maker and confusion-monger of all. The problem is this: when we talk about the values of the NHS (or of threats to them), what do we *mean*?

The words we typically use when we talk about the values of the NHS are 'needs', 'equality', 'equity' and 'fairness'. As we become better Europeans, we shall probably be adding words like 'solidarity'. The problem with these words is that their meaning is not clear. Nor is it clear to what they apply. For these two reasons it is not clear how they are to be implemented and whose jobs are on the line if they are not implemented.

Needs

The NHS is there to meet 'needs'. A need has to be for something. A need for something makes that thing necessary. Necessary for what? Suppose you answer, as some philosophers would, that *health* is needed (that is, is necessary) if people are to flourish and realize their potential as human beings. I think this is quite a plausible claim. But what implications does it have for the NHS? There are those who are gravely ill, or who are born with terrible congenital handicaps, whose ability to 'flourish' as humans, and to do so for any reasonable period, is terribly limited. There can be no doubt that they need *health*. And they may need many other things as well. But do they need health *care*? Do they need *medicine*? In many cases they don't – and for a cogent, if tragic, reason. There is nothing that the current technologies of medical care can do for their health. There may be palliative measures that could be taken with some benefit. If there are, they may well be needed. But medical care as we now know it is not a significant and necessary element for improving their health or helping them to flourish as well as they might.

You may want to go back a stage and say that what is really needed in such cases is appropriate measures to prevent the problem (or the birth) in the first place. And that too might be a sensible way of describing a claimed need for medical or health care, though it is likely to be a need for public rather than personal measures. It may also represent a claim that we (again collectively rather than individually) need environmental and other measures that are not related to health care – safer working environments, improved parenting skills, and the like.

Or, instead of going back, you may want to expand, as my last point suggests, to claim that what is needed, still based upon a desire for better health, is not a need for medicine, but rather for a battery of environmental measures. The need may even be for greater equality in the distribution of incomes and in the power and discretion that people have over their jobs and ways of working. I mention these two factors both because they have been identified as risk factors for ill-health in populations (and highly unequal distributions of it) (e.g. Wilkinson 1992; Marmot et al. 1991) and to illustrate the rather radical implications of a genuine attempt to develop a policy for *health*, merely a policy for *health care*.

Or you may want to go neither back nor to expand, but to go forward, to focus on the need for research: into the extension of the battery of effective medical procedures; into ways of improving technology transfer from the research world into the world of clinical practice; even research into research.

But, even granted all this, for cases of the sort I have mentioned, we have not established much about need for medical care that will help health authorities and medical professionals to make choices that are systematically based upon need. This has not deterred health services the world over from expensive and widespread interventions, sometimes extremely uncomfortable ones for the patients involved, carried out on people (often the frail and elderly) who desperately need health but who hardly need medicine at all. And why not, indeed? After all, that is how the medical professionals make their living. If they are paid, as in some systems, according to the medical acts performed (so much per assessment, so much per vagotomy, so much per multiple bypass operation, etc.) then the incentive to intervene expensively but fruitlessly in cases where the need for health is manifest becomes overwhelming. And why shouldn't it? Well, there is a very good reason why not. Because it is a waste of resources. Some people's health will not change for the better. Or not much for the better. Or, if a bit for the better, not for very long. And if that is how you are using your resources, then you will inevitably be denying resources to those for whom there really would be a marked improvement in health. Hip replacements, mostly for elderly women, have an absolutely dramatic effect on the quality of their lives. By anyone's standards they are highly effective in the majority of cases. Economists will tell you that they are also cheap per quality-adjusted additional year of life gained! There can be no doubt that they are needed. Yet the NHS for years left such manifest needs for health care languishing while resources were wasted elsewhere. And somehow, everyone (doctors, nurses, patients, managers, the general public) seems to believe that just because 'all possible' was done, the system is doing what it ought to do – meet needs. It just isn't true. But the myth is real. The myth is this: you should allocate health care resources according to the need for health! The truth is otherwise: if health (let us be more forceful and say 'maximum health') really is the objective, you should allocate resources according to the need for *health care* (or the need for other health-affecting activities, environments and so on).

But now consider the following. Suppose there are two people, Max and Moritz, both of whom are equally ill today and both of whom would gain equally in health terms from receiving the medical care appropriate to each case. Now suppose Max's treatment costs twice Moritz's. Therefore – mark this well – Max has the greater need (that is, he needs more health care). Would you want to allocate more resources to people like Max than to people like Moritz? Or, if you had to choose between treating Max or Moritz, would you necessarily want to choose Max? It is easy to make the contrary argument, because treating Moritz will produce the same health gain as treating Max, but there will be resources left over to treat other people. Those resources could be targeted either on achieving the highest further health gain possible or on achieving the maximum reduction feasible in the inequality of health and ill-health.

There are ways out of these conundrums. But this is not the place to enlarge upon them (see, e.g. Culyer and Wagstaff 1993; Culyer 1995). My point is to warn you about the rather remarkably contrary results that you can get once you try to put some sensible content into a word like 'need'. So we must be on guard when people use the language of 'need'. And we must sort out what idea of need should be used in the NHS.

Equality
Take 'equality'. Again, let us add some prepositions. Equality *of what*? One plainly cannot mean that everyone ought to receive the same amount of health care. Many people aren't ill at all and no one in their right mind would suggest that everyone ought to have an appendicectomy by, say, age 25, let alone chemotherapy for a non-existent cancer. This is not a daft as you may think. In the 1930s the American Child Health Association (1934) found, in a famous study, that 60 per cent of a sample of 1,000 New York children had not had a tonsillectomy (note the huge implied surgical intervention rate). In an experiment, the remaining 400 children were re-examined by school doctors, who selected 180 (45 per cent) as in need of tonsillectomy. The remaining 220 were then examined by a further group of doctors who found that a further 100 were in need of tonsillectomy. After three successive examinations, only 65 of the 1,000 received no recommendation for tonsillectomy. This, together with male circumcision, may be as near as one might ever get to the idea that surgery ought to be equally – literally equally – distributed!

But strict equality of this sort is plainly peculiar and I don't propose to discuss it further. Nearly everyone would agree, I suppose, that equality has to be tempered by some consideration of need. For example, the principle might be that equal need (say for a tonsillectomy) should (provided it really were a need!) be met by equal treatment. The qualifier 'provided it really were a need' is important and doubt about what is really necessary is probably the reason why even today in the NHS the rates of tonsillectomy vary hugely from area to area – from 7.5 per 10,000 at risk to 27.5. Similarly, at more aggregate levels of allocating resources, for example, when allocating central NHS resources to the health authorities in the UK, a strict allocation per capita would almost certainly be seen as unfair and inequitable, and for the same reason: it takes no account of the reasonable judgements that can be made about different needs in different areas. Such needs may, for example, be systematically related to the age and sex compositions of the populations of those areas. I do not say, you will note, the morbidity or mortality differences between areas, as I have already argued that ill-health as such may be a measure of the need for health, but it is not a measure of the need for health care.

Others will emphasize equality of opportunity or equal access. Here we confront some quite severe practical difficulties and some ethical ones as well. An example of a practical difficulty is that one's opportunity to receive health care, or its accessibility, depends not only on the cash price paid (whether zero or positive) and (if the price is positive) on one's income, but also on spatial factors (how distant one is from a clinic, surgery or hospital), the distribution of car ownership, whether one loses pay when one is absent from work to consult a doctor, and other similar factors. Measuring all these, even approximately, and trying to adjust resource availability accordingly is no mean task.

The ethical difficulty is more fundamental. Even if access were somehow made more equal for all, it does not follow that utilization would be more equal, even for those in equal need. After all, cultural factors and personal preferences also determine people's decisions to use health services, and these are certainly not equal for all. The inevitable consequence is that even equal access will result in different rates of use and, hence, different outcomes. But, if outcomes can differ, then you may end up *increasing* the inequality in the distribution of health and ill-health. Max and Moritz may have the same degree of ill-health. Let's suppose they now also need the same amount of health care. But if one benefits more than the other in terms of health, what was initially an equal distribution turns out to be an unequal one if they both receive the same amount of resources. So egalitarianism in one thing produces inequality in another. Moreover, equal access or opportunity does not imply *free* access. If everyone faced the same £10 consultation charge for visiting a GP, they would, at least in that respect, face an identical access cost. But would we agree that this was equitable? After all, the charge may deter the poor more than the rich and, since we know the poor to have worse health than the rich, the upshot may be to make the distribution of health in the community even worse. This highlights what I think is the death sentence on equality of access: it is sublimely unconcerned about outcomes.

The focus is wholly on inputs, and the outcomes, in terms of the health of people and its distribution amongst them, have no bearing at all on the resource distribution question. It seems to me, therefore, that the important thing about access and opportunity to consume health care is not so much that it ought to be equal but that it should be cheap. The reason for this is that, if resource distributions are to be related to need, people who are potentially in need have first to be assessed. *What* do they need? Without that initial contact with the GP and other professionals, the need for health care remains unknown. But it is this information that health service managers must possess if they are to be able to make the sorts of dispositions of resources in the NHS that would enable a principle like 'equal treatment for equal need' to work.

Effectiveness of medicine
I referred earlier to the ineffectiveness of some medical care. Recent reviews by authoritative bodies in the US and the UK have revealed the continuing use of procedures that do no good and of some that actually do harm (e.g. National Institutes of Health 1976, Department of Health 1992). One reason for this is that the results of research are not well disseminated amongst medical and other practitioners. Another is that a good many common and familiar procedures (as well as many new ones) have not been subject to critical scientific assessment for their effectiveness. Some of these are used to treat common problems that are not life-threatening and are cheap to treat. Glue ear is the most common cause of hearing impediment and is the reason for elective surgery in children. The surgical intervention rate in England is 4.7 per 1,000 children under the age of fifteen. Glue ear has been described as an 'epidemic' in *The Lancet*. Yet it seems that, because most glue ear cases resolve themselves spontaneously, the best strategy is 'watchful waiting', particularly since surgical intervention carries potentially serious risks to the patient (Effective Health Care 1992). Other interventions have built up strong public support. There is a fad for cholesterol screening, yet this will not make a contribution to lowering overall mortality from heart disease and should probably be actively *discouraged* (Effective Health Care 1993). Many common surgical procedures have outcomes that are in dispute, do little apparent good, and may do harm. The list includes cholecystectomy (surgical removal of the gall bladder), haemorrhoidectomy (surgical treatment of piles), hysterectomy, and, of course, tonsillectomy. These uncertainties probably account, at least in part, for the huge variations one can observe both internationally and within countries in intervention rates. Age-standardized rates for hysterectomy vary from 700 per 100,000 women in the US (mostly fee-per-item of surgery in this country of course) to 600 in Canada (which has free health care but still fee-for-service for the doctors), 450 in Australia, 250 in the UK and 110 in Norway (McPherson 1988). Which country is meeting needs

effectively? Within the UK there are dramatic variations in the rates of tonsillectomy, as has already been seen, and also in hysterectomy, prostatectomy and haemorrhoidectomy, where some rates are double others. One expert (McPherson 1988) in these matters has calculated that if eight common surgical procedures had been used in the UK with the vigour and enthusiasm for the knife of US surgeons, expenditure on them (the estimate was for 1986) would have more than doubled: from £176 million to £447 million.

The uncertainties about 'what works' in medicine should be distinguished from inherent uncertainty in particular cases, and variation in doctors' skills in diagnosis. One way in which medical and economic practices do differ lies in the possibility, in medicine, for subsequent reliable checking on the correctness of a diagnosis. A UK study in the early 1980s (Cameron and McGoogan 1981) found, on autopsies of patients who died while under treatment, that only 46.5 per cent were correct diagnoses; 39.8 per cent were wrong. The rate of missed conditions was 13.7 per cent. Of the wrong diagnoses, in 83 per cent of cases the cause of death was the true condition that had been misdiagnosed.

I am not, of course, trying to alarm. Nor am I belittling the work of doctors (one can rarely check on the economic diagnoses of economists, which are unlikely to be better than those of doctors and which can also have momentous consequences for the well-being of people). I have two points to make. First, we should not allow ourselves to be bamboozled by the apparent scientific glamour of medical science into supposing that it has all the answers, even to traditional medical questions. It should be more widely known that the major reductions in death rates from infectious diseases that have taken place in England, since records of cause of death began in 1837, occurred before medical interventions could possibly have had any impact. Take measles which, in 1900, was the largest infectious killer of children. Between 1850 and 1910 the death rate was about 1,100 per million children. From about 1915 mortality fell rapidly and continuously, becoming close to zero around 1960. But mass immunization dates only from around 1970. Mortality from measles is caused mainly by invasion by secondary organisms which have been treatable by drugs since 1935. But by 1935, 82 per cent of the decline in mortality between 1850 and 1971 had already taken place! (McKeown 1976). Historically, it is plain that there are other significant factors at work. In the case of measles the main one would seem to be nutritional improvements and possibly elimination of vitamin C deficiency in particular.

The second main point I want to make is that there is a good deal that can be done to improve medical decision-making, by encouraging knowledge-based clinical practice through disseminating research results and better ongoing medical education, through early training, through clinical audit, establishing clinical guidelines, and generally providing an environment in which practice is informed by knowledge about what works and what works for whom. These are far from trivial issues. Death rates from surgery are hugely variable from surgeon to surgeon and are not fully explicable by case complexity or patient-related factors. Operations performed only occasionally by a surgeon are less likely to be successful than those performed frequently. New techniques, like key-hole surgery, are most effectively applied by those who have had proper training by experts. The medical profession is characteristically defensive on all these matters. Information about them is not readily available, even to those like purchasing authorities who are least likely to misinterpret it and who, indeed, depend upon it for effective purchasing of health care for their client populations. This alone must be a powerful argument for the split created by the NHS reforms between purchasers and providers, for purchasers are charged with identifying the need for health care and with arranging for it to be met. Today there is, at last, a demand for information about 'what works' and its costs. And where there is a demand there is usually a supply response. It may take time but, so long as the purchasers keep up the pressure, it will eventually come.

Reprise

I have introduced these matters at some length because I do not believe that one can have an intelligent and purposeful discussion about any aspect of a health care system like the NHS unless one knows what challenges it faces (challenges such as the development of a knowledge-based service), unless one banishes from one's mind many of the myths that surround medicine and the NHS, and unless one is willing to address some fundamental issues about what one is trying to accomplish. The basic values, at the general level, seem clear. They are to use the available resources to maximum effect in improving the nation's health. I think we would all probably also agree that the system must be fair – but that pinning down exactly what we mean by this is an urgent task. I think we would all probably also agree that meeting needs is the NHS's main business; and identifying what we mean by needs and how we should fulfil them so that we could know reasonably well how we are actually performing is another soul-searching (or rather mind-searching) activity that is everyone's business. If we could be clear about these things we would be well on the way to getting a health service of which we really could be proud. Empty slogans about the NHS being 'the best in world' would become revealed for what they are – mere slogans. Political panic-mongering about 'privatizing' health care would also be shown to be empty posturing – after all, the aim is to get public purchasers in a position where they can see the needs and commission effective care to meet them in an equitable fashion. I call this 'demand-side socialism'. Whereas traditional socialism has tended to focus on the public ownership of the means of production and delivery, which we might call 'supply-side socialism' (though I don't mean to suggest that this focus has been exclusive), demand-side socialism focuses on the collective accountability of decision-makers on the demand side, with a more sceptical and pragmatic view being taken of the best (most efficient) means of delivery. Why should we, the public, care whether needs are met by private or public organizations – or, come to that, by for-profit or non-profit ones – provided that they meet the specifications of the public purchasers and can develop good working relations with them? We do not actually know what sorts of organization are best able to deliver effective care according to the rubrics set by public demanders such as health authorities and I doubt that we ever shall, in any general sense. We certainly shall not unless we open up the range of possibilities to purchasers to the fullest extent feasible. If it should turn out that private for-profit organizations produce a poor product at high cost, and that they are systematically worse employers than the public sector trusts, then they will not survive. Indeed, they may not get any NHS business in the first place. But their existence or non-existence is incidental. They may or may not be instrumental in the business of implementing the ideals of the NHS. I, for one, would not wish to prejudge the question for, were I to get it wrong, I would be compromising our ability to implement the values to which I have suggested we all subscribe.

What is to come

The chapters which follow explore the issues I have touched on here in greater detail. Each is by someone who has given a good deal of thought to the issues under discussion. Jeremy Hurst (Chapter 2) makes international comparisons, mostly between countries that share similar ideals for their health care systems but that have devised different (but apparently converging) means for attaining these ends. Robert Evans (Chapter 3) explores some fascinating aspects of the reasons for the systematic inequalities in health and ill-health that exist within societies (including our own) and the extent to which their correction is a matter to which health care has much to contribute. Is the NHS for ever doomed to pick up the pieces left because we have failed to understand the root causes of ill-health and to act on whatever understanding we do have? In his paper, Evans takes us into the realm of multidisciplinary insights into the 'pathways' through which the health of populations might be determined. Martin Chalkley and James Malcomson (Chapter 4) explore the extent to which contracting between purchasers and providers, whose separation is, as we have seen, a key element of the NHS reforms, is likely to deliver what is hoped from it and whether there is much hope that competition between providers can deliver more cost-effective care. Cam Donaldson (Chapter 5) takes up the principle of need as a criterion for allocating NHS resources through the purchasing strategies of health authorities. David Mayston (Chapter 6) examines the way in which trusts (especially hospitals and community services) respond in their investment and manpower decisions to the rather peculiar constraints that the 'managed' internal market currently imposes on them. Alistair McGuire (Chapter 7) investigates the possibilities for insurance models in the finance of the NHS, particularly in the context of their possible use as a means of correcting the so-called underfunding of the NHS. Finally, Julian Le Grand (Chapter 8) takes up the great theme of equity and fairness, especially as it confronts purchasers.

It will be clear from what I have said that my own belief is that, despite ambiguities about the values that ought to be embodied in the NHS, the reforms are more of a challenge than a threat. Indeed, they are quite specifically a challenge to health authorities and health service providers to be more explicit about their values and to develop their strategies in accordance with them. They may, of course, fail miserably. But I am a moderate optimist and will settle for something better than we have had, even if it is not perfect. But there is another challenge which is less one for the health services than for society as a whole. This challenge is first to understand better the causes of illness and incapacity and, second, to use this understanding to build a healthier society. The NHS is not really a *health* service. Nor has it ever been. It is a *sickness* service. The more fundamental challenge to us all is to develop a health policy that will include the appropriate role of medical and social care within it, but which will also transcend these familiar elements by embracing other policies suggested by the sort of research programme outlined by Robert Evans in his paper.

Do not expect a consistent message! I doubt that the differences you may detect between the authors in this book could be attributable to any of the 'gaps' in understanding with which I began. They are more likely to reflect what I hope I have established as a fact, that we remain, despite nearly fifty years of rhetoric, in largely uncharted conceptual and empirical waters. Also do not expect the authors to stick only to science. The interweaving of ethics and science is too thorough for that. But watch out for one masquerading as the other! Above all, I hope that our contribution to this festival of science will help readers to set science in its place in policy debate. It is crucial but it is not enough. It is necessary but it is not sufficient. I hope also that the book will enable the reader to see better the place of health care in health policy. It too is crucial but not enough. It too is necessary but not sufficient. In an age when we all know so much more about so much less, a successful health policy depends, I suggest, on more of us trying to be renaissance people, asking deeper questions and answering them from wider perspectives. A wider public needs to become involved in these debates. To get such an involvement is one purpose of this collection of essays.

References

American Child Health Association (1934), *The Pathway to Correction in Physical Defects*, New York: ACHA.

Cameron, H.M. and McGoogan, E. (1981), 'A prospective study of 1,152 hospital autopsies, Parts I and II', *Journal of Pathology*, **133**, 273–83, 285–300.

Culyer, A.J. (1995), 'Need: the idea won't do – but we still need it', *Social Science and Medicine*, **40**, 727–30.

Culyer, A.J. and Wagstaff, A. (1993), 'Equity and equality in health and health care', *Journal of Health Economics*, **12**, 431–58.

Department of Health (1992), *Assessing the Effects of Health Technologies: Principles, Practice, Proposals*, London: Department of Health.

Department of Health and Social Security (1980), *Inequalities in Health* (The Black Report), Report of a Research Working Group Chaired by Sir Douglas Black, London: DHSS.

Effective Health Care (1992), *The Treatment of Persistent Glue Ear in Children*, no. 4, York: University of York.

Effective Health Care (1993), *Cholesterol: Screening and Treatment*, no. 6, York: University of York.

HM Government (1989), *Working for Patients*, CM555, London: HMSO.

Marmot, M.G., Davey Smith, G., Stansfield, S., Patel, C., North, F., Head, J., White, I., Brunner, E. and Feeney, A. (1991), 'Health inequalities among British civil servants: the Whitehall II study', *The Lancet*, **8384**, 1002–6.

McKeown, T. (1976), *The Modern Rise of Population*, London: Edward Arnold.

McPherson, K. (1988), *Variations in Hospitalisation Rates: Why and How to Study Them*, London: King's Fund Institute.

National Institutes of Health Trials Committee (1976), *Clinical Trials and the Public's Interest*, Bethesda: NIH.

Wilkinson, R.G. (ed.) (1986), *Class and Health, Research and Longitudinal Data*, London: Tavistock.

Wilkinson, R.G. (1992), 'Income distribution and life expectancy', *British Medical Journal*, **304**, 165–8.

2   The NHS reforms in an international context

Jeremy Hurst

Introduction

This chapter places the recent reforms to the UK's health services in an international context.

As befits a paper prepared for a festival of science, it is concerned with questions of classification and causation: with exploring whether some designs of health care system perform better than others. An attempt is made to separate normative questions, about ends, from positive questions, about means.

An international perspective has been adopted because in economics, unlike the natural sciences, it is usually impracticable to conduct controlled experiments, especially with whole systems. International comparisons provide economists with one of their few opportunities to observe 'natural' experiments with systems from which they can try to draw conclusions about causation and performance.

The main message of this chapter is that the recent reforms to the National Health Service (NHS) in the UK – both what was changed and what was not changed – fit into a pattern of convergence between health care systems. There have long been signs of growing agreement among countries about the objectives of health care systems. Now there are signs – albeit weak ones – of growing agreement about means.

This chapter is based on a recent study carried out for the Organization for Economic Cooperation and Development (OECD) of the reform of health care in seven OECD countries (OECD 1992). It is also informed by the findings which have emerged from a further study of health care reform in the remaining seventeen OECD countries (OECD 1994).

The recent reforms to the National Health Service

The reforms to the NHS which took place in 1990 and 1991 (HMSO 1989) were as remarkable for what they left unchanged in the NHS as for what they altered. Unchanged were: universal access to comprehensive medical care financed out of general taxation; and services provided to patients mainly free of charge. There were four main changes.

1. A new contract was introduced for GPs which made patients' choice of GP easier and introduced new incentives for GPs to offer services such as preventive care and minor surgery.
2. In the hospital sector a separation was introduced – mediated by contracts – between district health authorities as purchasers and hospitals as providers.
3. Large GP practices were given the opportunity to control part of the funds available for hospital to allow them to purchase outpatient and some surgical inpatient services on behalf of their patients (GP 'fundholding').
4. Finally, well-managed hospitals were given the opportunity to become self-governing trusts with more autonomy than the directly managed units they replaced.

Together, the last three changes involved: the introduction of an 'internal' or 'quasi' market into the NHS; an increase in delegated authority compared with the previous more centralized system; and a potential for a shift away from 'command and control' regulation towards regulation based on promoting competition among providers.

The objectives of health care policy

Both the old and the new elements of the reformed NHS can be seen as consistent with a list of health care policy objectives which, it can be argued, have been adopted explicitly or implicitly by most OECD members. These objectives, quoting from OECD (1992), are:

Adequacy and equity in access to care: there should be some minimum of health care available to all citizens and treatment should be in accordance with need; at least in the publicly financed sector.

Income protection: patients should be protected from payments for health care which threaten income sufficiency and the payment for protection should be linked to patients' ability to pay. This will involve at least three types of transfer: insurance (the need for care is unpredictable); saving (the elderly use more services than the young) and income redistribution (the sick are often the poor).

Macroeconomic efficiency: health care should consume an appropriate fraction of the Gross Domestic Product (GDP).

Microeconomic efficiency: a mix of services should be chosen which maximizes a combination of health outcome and consumer satisfaction, given the available resources. In addition, costs should be minimized for any given service. There should also be a search for technological and organizational change which improves benefits for given costs.

Freedom of choice for consumers: freedom of choice should be available in public as well as private sector arrangements.

Appropriate autonomy for providers: doctors and other providers should be given the maximum freedom consistent with attainment of the above objectives – especially in matters of medical and organizational innovation.

The nature of the 1990–91 reforms to the NHS suggests that, at least in the government's view, the pre-reform NHS was performing well on the first three of these objectives but less well on the last three.

Alternative subsystems for financing and delivering health care

What international differences are there in the means which have been adopted for pursuing these objectives? Analysts hoping to make international comparisons of health care systems are faced with what appears, at first glance, to be a bewildering diversity of health care institutions in different countries. However, once the superficial differences in nomenclature and organizational arrangements have been cleared away, it becomes apparent that most health care systems are made up from different mixtures of a few simple building blocks or subsystems. My suggestion (following Evans 1981) is that there are about eight such building blocks found in the OECD group of countries. I shall describe and discuss six of these before using them to analyse reforms in a number of OECD countries. Two other building blocks, varieties of health maintenance organizations, are covered in the OECD (1992) volume.

Each building block (except the first) is made up of financial and service delivery relationships for health care between five main sets of actors:

- consumers/patients;
- 'first-level providers', such as the GP, who can be approached directly by the patient;
- 'second-level providers', such as the hospital inpatient department, access to which is controlled by doctors;
- 'third party funding bodies', such as insurers or government-sponsored 'purchasers' which finance health care indirectly; and
- the government, in its capacity as regulator of the system.

Private, direct purchase of health care

The simplest and historically earliest arrangement for purchasing health care is the straightforward private market depicted in Figure 2.1. Consumers (patients) are shown on the left. First- and second-level providers are on the right. The providers are shown as multiple to indicate that there is competition between them. Solid lines between the boxes denote health service flows. Dotted lines denote financial flows. Wavy lines denote referral flows. It is assumed that patients pay directly for health care, by fee per item or per service.

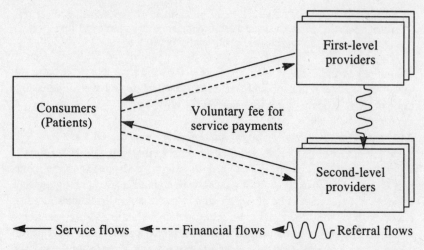

Service flows ◄---- Financial flows ◄〰〰 Referral flows

Figure 2.1   Voluntary, out-of-pocket payment for health care

It is assumed that such a market would be regulated in two ways: self-regulation by the caring professions and general market regulation by the government.

All OECD countries still rely on this basic mechanism for delivering health care to some extent. For example, non-prescribed medicines are usually provided and marketed in this way.

How does this simple system perform against the health policy objectives set out above? It will not perform well in terms of adequacy and equity. Access to care will be rationed by ability to pay. The poor will find access to care difficult or impossible. Even relatively affluent families may be denied access or be financially ruined if the breadwinner is incapacitated by serious illness. However, for those patients who can afford care the prospects for efficiency are good. Patients will be quality- and cost-conscious when choosing their provider, which will ensure that there are incentives for suppliers to offer value for money. However, because there will be asymmetry of knowledge in medical matters, consumers can be vulnerable to poor treatment and overcharging. It is the role of professional and government regulation to control that. Even this simple market is likely to require regulation and management.

Private health insurance with reimbursement of patients
Figure 2.2 depicts a private health care market with the introduction of competitive private health insurance of the kind where the insurer reimburses the patient in whole or in part for medical care bills. Note that in its pure form reimbursement insurance involves no contact between insurers and providers. Medical bills are still paid by patients.

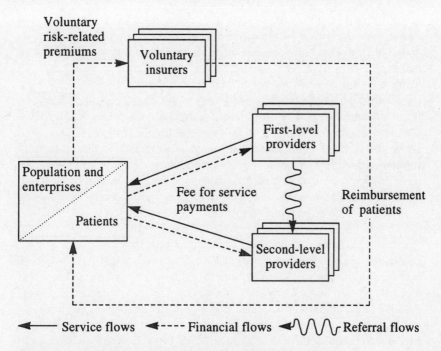

Figure 2.2   Voluntary insurance with reimbursement of patients

Such 'reimbursement' insurance is found in many OECD countries. It is still the dominant form of private health insurance in the US and in the UK, although it is now undergoing modifications in both countries.

The introduction of private insurance into the simple health care market will enable risks to be spread. Affluent individuals, if insured, need no longer fear the financial consequences of catastrophic acute illness.

For the poor and chronically sick, however, the availability of insurance will be of little help. The poor will not be able to afford it and the chronically sick will find that in a competitive market insurance is refused or premiums are loaded against them.

Moreover, the introduction of private insurance of the reimbursement type will have a devastating effect on efficiency. Once a third party has accepted the responsibility of paying, in whole or in part, for all 'reasonable' medical care, both patient and doctor have a reduced incentive to economize on treatments. Such arrangements reward the providers who offer the most lavish care. Medical care is no different from any other service. As its volume per capita rises it is subject to diminishing returns as more trivial conditions are treated with less effective interventions. The aim should be to balance marginal benefits against marginal costs. A reimbursement mechanism removes all or part of the cost element from this equation and makes it almost certain that care will be taken beyond the point where marginal benefit equals marginal cost. That will seem rational to both patient and doctor if bills are being paid by a third party and additional needs (however small) are still being met. But it would not be rational for a fully informed and fully cost-conscious patient. The result is likely to be a cycle of escalating claims and fees. Although this will result in rising premiums, which may lead to some consumer resistance, it is likely that any equilibrium will be reached well above the level of expenditure that would arise under the first model described. If there is tax relief for insurance premiums, achievement of equilibrium itself may be in doubt. Under reimbursement insurance, there will still be incentives for providers to minimize costs but price competition among providers is likely to be replaced by quality competition.

Public health insurance with reimbursement of patients
One of the great social discoveries of the late nineteenth and early twentieth centuries in Europe was the possibility of public insurance for sickness and other threats to lifetime earnings for workers and their dependants. It is possible to set up one financial risk pool to which all members of a community, occupation or industry are required to contribute, according to ability to pay, and from which the sick are authorized to draw according to need. Such insurance can be set up on reimbursement lines as in the previous model. That is, private provision of medical care can be left undisturbed with patients claiming retrospectively for all or part of any reasonable medical care bill. Figure 2.3 depicts such an arrangement. It is identical to Figure 2.2 except that the insurance box is shown as single, rather than multiple, to denote a single public, risk-pooling insurer. National health insurance in France in the 1950s approximated to such an arrangement.

Although a system of public reimbursement for medical care bills can meet the objectives of adequacy and equity, it is unlikely to meet the objective of macroeconomic efficiency. As in the private reimbursement model, neither patient nor doctor will have very much incentive to economize on medical care. Total health expenditure is likely to rise unacceptably rapidly for the public purse. Moreover, to the extent that health care is financed by payroll taxes, high expenditure is likely to discourage employment. To some extent the growth of health expenditure may be restrained by introducing cost-sharing by patients. However, if such charging becomes high enough to deter use significantly, it is likely to undermine the adequacy and equity objectives of the scheme.

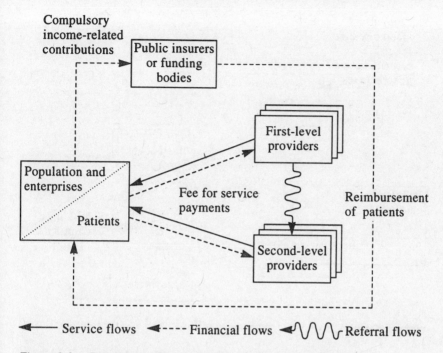

Service flows ◄---- Financial flows ◄∿∿Referral flows

Figure 2.3 Compulsory insurance with reimbursement of patients

The public 'integrated' model

One solution to this dilemma has been for the government to take over the provision as well as the financing of medical care. Doctors and pharmacists can be employed on salary in the public sector. Hospitals may be taken into public ownership and given fixed, annual global budgets to cover their running costs. That means that there is no longer any requirement for patients to pay medical care bills – care is provided free of charge to patients when it is needed. Such a system is depicted in Figure 2.4. Note that there is now a direct connection between the funding body and the providers. Now, the providers' boxes are single to denote that in its pure form this model will lack consumer choice. Patients will be assigned to providers. The decision on the total level of health expenditure in such a system becomes the responsibility of the government.

Such public, 'integrated' arrangements were the standard model in the former Soviet Union and in Eastern Europe before the collapse of communism. They were also popular in many Western European countries including Scandinavia. They were the basis for the financing and delivery of hospital care in the UK before the reforms of 1991.

Such a system, if well run, is quite capable of meeting the objectives of adequate and equitable treatment for all. It is also quite capable of meeting

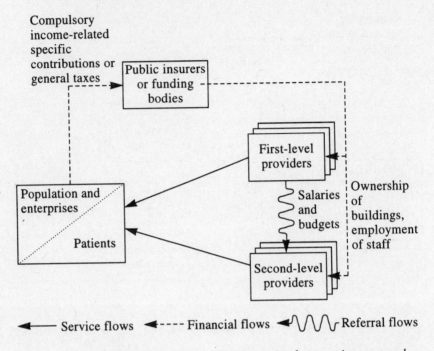

Figure 2.4   *Compulsory insurance with integration between insurers and providers*

the macroeconomic goal, provided the government has the political courage to control health expenditure. Also, integrated models are well designed to pursue public health goals and, hence, preventive strategies. Where the system is likely to fall down is in the areas of microeconomic efficiency, consumer satisfaction and appropriate provider autonomy. The integrated system contains perverse financial incentives. It is likely to suffer from what has been dubbed 'the efficiency trap'. If providers serve customers well they are likely to be rewarded by more work, not more money. If they perform poorly or divert resources to ends of their own choosing, they are likely to be rewarded by a quiet life and will not necessarily suffer financially. That happens because, unlike as in all the previous models, money does not follow the patient. Although it is possible to have patient choice in the integrated model it is unlikely to be effective in encouraging efficiency so long as money does not follow the patient. Integrated systems tend to be characterized by queues and an impersonal service. Their patients tend to behave like grateful supplicants rather than empowered consumers. Similarly, integrated systems tend to contain poor local incentives for reducing costs. High-level budget-setters may respond to efficiency gains by taking away savings and to inefficiency by increasing grants. The government may try to avoid such mistakes but is seldom likely to have the information to do so. Its sole regulatory weapon is 'command and control' which is likely to be inimical to appropriate autonomy among providers. At their best, such systems can run well where professionals and managers are competent and dedicated, and public expectations are low. At their worst, such systems can be 'captured' by the providers and may even become corrupted – for example by 'under-the-table' payments from patients to providers as in some of the former systems in Eastern Europe.

The public contract model

The perverse financial incentives in the public integrated model may be tackled by: introducing separation between the public funding bodies and the providers; by introducing contracts with fee-for-service or capitation payments; by granting more autonomy to the providers and by allowing patient choice of first-level provider and patient/doctor choice of second-level provider. Such a public 'contract' system can be run like a market rather than a bureaucracy. This system is depicted in Figure 2.5. Note that the boxes for the providers have become multiple. Care may still be provided free of charge to

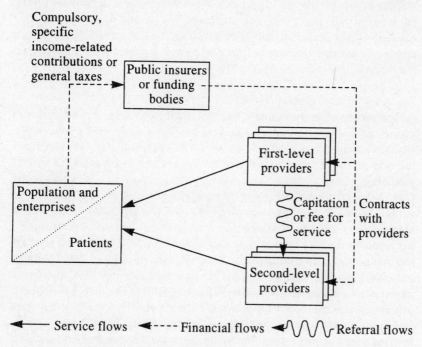

Figure 2.5   Compulsory insurance with insurer/provider contracts

the patient, and public funding bodies can, if they are determined, still impose overall budgetary constraints on providers.

Such public contractual arrangements for health care are familiar in the UK because they have always formed the basis for the financing arrangements for family practitioners, including GPs, under the NHS. They have been established more widely in countries such as Belgium, France, Germany, the Netherlands, Canada and Japan.

Public contract systems are just as capable as integrated systems of meeting adequacy and equity objectives. They can, through budgetary controls, be made to meet macroeconomic objectives. They seem to offer better prospects than the integrated model for microeconomic efficiency driven by consumer and doctor choice, because money follows the patient, which means that payments to providers tend to be performance-related. They also give providers appropriate autonomy. Regulation can, if desired, take the form of a mixture of command and control, via the public-funding bodies, and pro-competitive regulation of the providers. The former would allow, say, public health goals to be pursued. The latter can be used to foster efficiency and responsiveness to consumers.

That is not to say that public contract models have always been without problems. Historically, the price exacted by the medical profession for setting up such models was often free choice of any doctor by the patient; the freedom of any doctor to join the scheme; and fee-for-service. The first two provisions relegated the funding bodies to passive payers and the latter built in an upward pressure on expenditure.

The public, double contract model

A 'limitation' of the last three models is that the consumer has no choice of insurer or funding body. Policy-makers have now developed a new, public 'double-contract' model which allows for consumer choice between funding bodies. In the 'pure' version of the model, the funding bodies will be public or private insurers. In a hybrid version, they can be fundholding GPs. To make it public, this model requires a device such as a central fund which can levy compulsory contributions from the population according to ability to pay and pay out risk-related, transferable premiums or capitation payments to funding bodies on behalf of the insured. The insured are then free to contract with the insurer or funder of their choice. To the extent that premiums/vouchers can be adjusted for risk, the insurers will have reduced incentives to pursue risk selection. The central fund can also be used as a capping device, to help to ensure cost containment. This model is depicted in Figure 2.6. It is particularly suited to countries which already have a large private insurance sector and a desire to incorporate it within a public system.

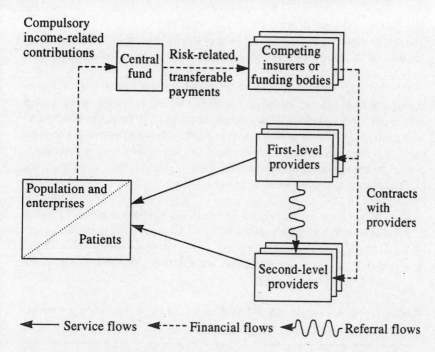

Figure 2.6   Compulsory insurance with competition among both insurers and providers

This model has been adopted recently in Switzerland and in parts of the former Soviet Union. It has been under discussion in the Netherlands – which has a large private insurance sector – for some time but by mid-1995 had not been fully implemented there. In essence, it formed the basis for President Clinton's 1993 proposals for the reform of health care in the US (The White House 1993) which were rejected by Congress. The GP fundholding variant has been adopted in a limited way in the UK.

The capabilities of this new model have yet to be demonstrated by prolonged use. On paper, it seems to offer greater flexibility and potential for organizational innovation than the public single-contract model. However, it may be less suited to the pursuit of public health goals. Also, since, in practice, it is difficult to adjust payments to funding bodies for risk, risk selection may remain a problem requiring regulation. Nevertheless, many observers feel that GP fundholding has been the most dynamic and successful part of the new NHS internal market (Glennerster et al. 1994; National Audit Office 1994).

Health care reforms in selected OECD countries
The classification system developed above can be used to categorize the main features of the health care systems in OECD countries and the major structural reforms to them.

Most of the countries have systems which represent mixtures of two or three of the subsystems described above. For example, the system in the UK before the 1991 reforms can be categorized as a mixture of the public contract system for ambulatory care and the public integrated system for hospital care. Superimposed on those was a small, private reimbursement and out-of-pocket payment system for private medicine.

The reforms to the NHS can be categorized as:

- a move from the integrated model to the contract model for hospital and community health services;
- a partial and evolving adoption of a variant of the double-contract model for part of hospital and community health service care, in the shape of GP fundholding.

Table 2.1   Main components of health care systems in ten OECD countries, circa 1990

	Public spending as a percentage of total health expenditure 1990	Public finance of primary medical care	Public finance of hospital care
Belgium	89	R&C	C
France	74	R&C	C&I
W. Germany	72	C	C
Netherlands	71	C	C
Ireland	75	C	I
Norway	95	I&C	I
Spain	80	I	I&C
Sweden	80	I	I
UK	84	C	I
US	42	R&C	R,C&I

R = reimbursement
C = contract
I = integrated

A summary of the main characteristics of the health care systems of ten OECD countries in 1990, using this classification system, is given in Table 2.1. The first column shows the public share of total health expenditure. The last two columns show the main financing/delivery models adopted for primary medical care and hospital care, respectively, in each country.

All the systems except that of the US were dominated by public spending on health care in 1990. The first four countries in the table – Belgium, France, Germany and the Netherlands – relied mainly on the public contract model. Belgium and France had vestiges of the reimbursement model in ambulatory care. The next five countries – Ireland, Norway, Spain, Sweden and the UK – were dominated mainly by the public integrated model, at least for hospital care. The last country – the US – was dominated by private spending, mainly via the reimbursement model, although by 1994 an estimated 20 per cent of the US population was enrolled with health maintenance organizations. The public sector of health care in the US was unusually complex with a mix of mechanisms for different sectors of the population such as Medicare (mainly reimbursement), Medicaid (partly contract) and the Veterans Affairs Medical Program (mainly integrated).

It is convenient to discuss the reforms to health care systems in these ten countries under three main headings, which have been designed to summarize the health policy objectives set out earlier in this chapter:

- adequacy and equity of access to medical care;
- macroeconomic efficiency; and
- microeconomic efficiency.

Reforms aimed at improving adequacy and equity
For several decades, the predominant trend in OECD countries has been towards increasing public coverage for health care risks. Hence, it is unsurprising that at the time of the 1991 reforms to the NHS, the UK continued to adhere to the principle of universal public coverage, which had been established in the UK in 1948.

During the 1980s, Spain made its scheme universal and the Netherlands announced her intention to proceed to universal health coverage against all major risks as part of the 'Dekker' plan. In 1994 Switzerland adopted national health insurance. Dwarfing these changes is the fact that recently both the US and Turkey have announced an aspiration to proceed towards universal health insurance. These two countries are the last in the OECD (1993 membership) with significant gaps in health insurance coverage which affect the poor.

Reforms aimed at improving macroeconomic efficiency

Following the decade of the 1970s, when many countries experienced cost explosions in health care, most OECD countries took steps to gain more control over their health expenditure in the 1980s.

The discussion above suggests that countries which rely on the integrated and contract models will find it easier to control public expenditure on health than countries which rely on the reimbursement model.

Table 2.2 shows the experience of the ten countries in terms of changes to the health expenditure share of their GDPs in the 1970s and 1980s. Three main conclusions can be drawn:

1. All these countries except the US reduced the rate of growth of the health expenditure shares of their GDPs in the 1980s compared with the 1970s.
2. The US, which relied mainly on the reimbursement model, increased its share.
3. The two countries which reduced their GDP share farthest, in absolute terms, in the 1980s, Ireland and Sweden, both relied on the integrated model. However Germany, which relies on the contract model, also reduced its share by one percentage point.

The probable explanation for the success of the four countries with mainly contract models in controlling expenditure in the 1980s is that all four introduced global budgets for hospital services in that decade, and Germany introduced global budgets for primary medical care services a few years earlier. The Netherlands already paid its GPs by capitation which probably helped it to contain costs compared with Belgium and France which paid primary care doctors by fee-for-service. Ireland abandoned fee-for-service payments for primary care doctors in 1989 and joined the UK and the Netherlands in paying by capitation.

The UK has long had a reputation for tight control of NHS health expenditure and it maintained that reputation in the 1980s. What is clear from Table 2.2 is that neighbouring countries in Western Europe increasingly joined the UK, many of them reforming their health care systems to do so.

On the whole, the experience in Western Europe was borne out elsewhere in the OECD. Over half of the remaining countries for which we have data reduced their health expenditure shares in the 1980s compared with the 1970s.

President Clinton's proposals of 1993 for radical reform of the American health care system gave prominence to measures to control costs by '...increasing competition in health care, reducing administrative costs and imposing budget discipline'. It was envisaged that the government would take

Table 2.2   Health expenditure shares of GDP

	Health expenditure as a percentage share of GDP			Percentage change in health expenditure share	
	1970	1980	1990	1970–80	1980–90
Belgium	4.1*	6.6	7.6	61*	15
France	5.8	7.6	8.8	31	16
Germany	5.9	8.4	8.3	42	−1
Netherlands	6.0	8.0	8.2	33	3
Ireland	5.6	9.2	7.0	64	−24
Norway	5.0	6.6	7.4	32	12
Spain	3.7	5.6	6.6	51	18
Sweden	7.2	9.4	8.6	31	−9
UK	4.5	5.8	6.2	29	7
US	7.4	9.2	12.4	24	35

* The 1970 figure may be underestimated.

Source: OECD (1993), *Health Systems: Facts and Trends.*

powers to limit the rate of growth of insurance premiums if the first two of these measures failed to contain costs (The White House 1993). Interestingly enough, in the same year that Congress rejected these plans, large US employers experienced an unprecedented 2 per cent fall in health care costs per employee, probably because so many shifted the health insurance contracts for their workers towards health maintenance organizations and other forms of managed care (*Financial Times*, 15 February 1995). Private contract and integrated models have not been discussed in this chapter but are described in OECD (1992). It remains to be seen whether such forms of private health insurance can bring about a sustained reduction in the rate of growth of health expenditure in the US.

Reforms aimed at improving microeconomic efficiency
In the late 1980s and early 1990s a growing list of countries, especially those with public integrated health care systems, adopted or moved towards structural reforms aimed at improving microeconomic efficiency.

Several countries with integrated systems adopted public contract or double public contract systems. Sweden and New Zealand joined the UK in

separating purchasers and providers and setting up internal markets. Following the reunification of Germany, measures were taken swiftly to set about
restoring the former Bismarckian contract model in the area occupied by the
former German Democratic Republic. Some of the other countries of Eastern
Europe looked towards Germany, France and the Netherlands in replacing
their integrated models. The former Soviet Union has adopted various experiments with the double-contract model.

The reason for these changes was a belief that more market-based approaches would make public integrated systems both more effective – especially in respect of consumer responsiveness – and more productive, lessen-
ing demands on governments for even greater health expenditure. This
'perestroika' in health care in the late 1980s can be associated with the
contemporary disillusionment with central planning and state provision in
whole economies.

But is there any *evidence* that integrated health care systems embedded in
mixed Western economies were less efficient than contract systems? Unfortunately, although international data on health system inputs are plentiful, data
on health service outcomes are scarce or of poor quality. The following
analysis is based on an attempt to assemble input and outcome data for our
ten selected countries. Clearly, it is hazardous to try to compare three different types of health care system across so few countries. Nevertheless, it is
possible to check whether the available evidence, such as it is, is grossly
inconsistent, or not, with the hypotheses about the performance of the different systems set out above.

Table 2.3 records one measure of input – expenditure per head in US$
(column 1) – and four measures of outcome – perinatal mortality; patients'
average waiting time to see a specialist after referral by a GP ('outpatient'
waiting time); patients' average inpatient waiting time; and a measure of
general satisfaction with the health care system (columns 2–5). The countries
are grouped into three main categories according to their dominant financing
and delivery models, as before.

It must be pointed out that some of the data in the table leave much to be
desired. The figures on health expenditure have been adjusted for general
purchasing power parity (PPP) exchange rates but not for medical care PPP
exchange rates (which in mid-1995 were still not available in a reliable
form). Definitions of perinatal mortality may differ slightly between countries. The data on average waiting times derive from a survey of 1,500 non-
randomly selected GPs in fifteen European countries each of whom recorded data on 30 consecutive patient referrals (RCGP 1992). The data on
satisfaction derive from a series of linked opinion surveys, each involving
about 1,000 respondents, collected in eleven countries in various years
between 1988 and 1991 (Blendon et al. 1990, 1991). There are some

Table 2.3   One measure of input and four measures of outcome for ten OECD countries

	1 Health expenditure per capita in US$, 1989[1]	2 Perinatal mortality rate, 1989[2]	3 Mean outpatient waiting time, days, circa 1989[3]	4 Mean inpatient waiting time, days, circa 1989[3]	5 Percentage satisfied with health care system, circa 1989[4]
Belgium	1,153	1.02[5]	7.5	n.a.	n.a.
France	1,415	0.89	6.3	n.a.	41
Germany	1,412	0.64	6.9	11.2	41
Netherlands	1,176	0.96	10.8	18.8	47
Ireland	651	0.99	27.4	n.a.	n.a.
Norway	1,128	0.76	33.7	13.1	n.a.
Spain	682	0.88	12.0	21.9	21
Sweden	1,390	0.65	n.a.	n.a.	32
UK	912	0.83	36.3	29.6	27
US	2,362	0.96	n.a.	n.a.	10

Notes:
1. At GDP, purchasing power parity exchange rates, source: OECD (1993), *Health Systems, Facts & Trends.*
2. Percent of live and still births, source: OECD, as above.
3. Source: RCGP (1992), *The European Study of Referrals from Primary to Secondary Care,* London.
4. Proportion of individuals in a random sample survey who agreed with the statement, 'On the whole, the health care system works pretty well, and only a few changes are necessary to make it work better'. Sources: Blendon et al. (1990 and 1991).
5. 1987.

significant gaps in the columns of figures where data are not available (n.a.).

The table reveals substantial differences both in health expenditure per capita and in performance. Differences in health expenditure per capita are explained mainly by differences in GDP per capita. That is, health expenditure rises approximately linearly with GDP per capita, although in 1989 the UK lay somewhat below a regression line fitted between the two (Schieber et al. 1991).

Starting with health outcome, there is little if any sign of an association between perinatal mortality, one of the few measures we have of health outcome, and either health expenditure per capita or the type of health care system. The UK performed slightly better than the average country in the group of ten. The US had approximately the same perinatal mortality as Ireland, despite having nearly four times its level of health expenditure per capita. Integrated systems seem to perform at least as well as contract or reimbursement systems in this respect.

Moving on to waiting times, there are marked signs that queues are longer in countries which had integrated hospital systems in 1990. For example, the UK had the longest outpatient and inpatient waiting times among the ten countries. It is less clear that there is an association between waiting times and health expenditure per capita. For example, Norway had long outpatient waiting times despite its high level of health expenditure per capita.

Turning to consumer satisfaction, there are marked signs that general satisfaction with health care systems was lower in countries with integrated systems than in countries with contract systems. Lower still was satisfaction in the US – presumably because of its combination of lack of cover for many and high costs for all. Even if we put aside the US, there is little evidence of an association between satisfaction and health expenditure per capita. Sweden had the third highest level of health care spending among the nine European countries but its reported satisfaction level was well below that of France, Germany and the Netherlands.

These findings on satisfaction have been echoed by a regular survey of consumer opinion *within* the UK. This survey suggests that public satisfaction is greater with general practice (contract model) than with hospital services, especially outpatient services (integrated model). Moreover, following the reforms, satisfaction with the NHS has been rising, reversing the trend of the 1980s (SCPR 1991, 1994).

In view of the patchy nature of the available outcome data, and the fact that most of the ten systems are to some extent a mixture of subsystems, each with different incentives, it is not possible to draw any very firm conclusions. However, it could be said, in summary form, that the evidence is not inconsistent with the hypothesis that integrated systems are less successful than contract systems in raising consumer satisfaction and in limiting queues.

In addition to moves from the integrated to the contract and double-contract model, there were also moves towards microeconomic reforms in countries which relied mainly upon contract and reimbursement models. Germany introduced measures encouraging more competition between hospitals and between pharmaceutical companies supplying drugs under national health insurance. It introduced competition between sickness funds in 1993. Switzerland adopted a version of the double-contract model in 1994. And, as we have seen, both the Netherlands and the US developed plans for adopting the double-contract model. There was no inclination in either of these two countries to lessen their reliance on markets in health care. Rather, they envisaged preserving the scope for competition within extended public schemes. Both plans, however, ran into insurmountable political opposition, stemming partly from the insurers and providers who would be affected by them.

Conclusion

The main theme of this paper has been that the recent reforms to the health care system in the UK fit into a pattern of convergence between health care systems among OECD countries.

There seems to be underlying, if not overt, agreement about the objectives of most OECD health care systems: adequate and equitable services for all; macroeconomic efficiency; and microeconomic efficiency based on consumer choice and appropriate provider autonomy.

Now there are signs – though faint ones – of a growing agreement about means. These means include: public health insurance or funding to cover all, or all who cannot otherwise afford insurance cover; political control of the overall level of health expenditure; and the use of managed, market or quasi-market mechanisms to motivate and channel providers and, in some systems, insurers.

In terms of the categories of health care financing and delivery system developed in this paper, that means a convergence on the public contract and public double-contract models from, on the one hand, the private reimbursement model and, on the other hand, the public integrated model.

The UK reforms fit into this pattern both in terms of what was changed and what was not changed. We have kept our universal cover and firm political control over health expenditure. We have relinquished our former reliance on integrated public provision and central planning in favour of a managed 'internal' market (contract). We are also developing GP fundholding (double-contract). Meanwhile, countries like the US have considered adopting universal health insurance together with public control of health expenditure while retaining their competitive markets for health care and health insurance (double-contract).

It would be wrong to exaggerate the degree or the speed of convergence between OECD health care systems. There remains significant diversity among them, especially on matters of detail. Moreover, some of the potential convergence has been stalled by the political process.

Furthermore, there remain a number of unanswered questions about the effectiveness of different designs of health care system, especially the relatively untried 'pure' double-contract model. In the UK, two outstanding questions are: the final role of GP fundholding in the scheme of things; and the appropriate balance between management and competition in the new internal market. It is clear that the debate over health care financing and organization did not come to an end in the UK in April 1991. Nor has it come to an end among OECD countries as a whole.

References

Bartlett, W. and Le Grand, J. (1994), 'The Performance of Trusts' in Robinson, R. and Le Grand, J. (eds), *Evaluating the NHS Reforms*, London: King's Fund Institute.

Blendon, R.J. et al. (1990), 'Satisfaction with Health Systems in Ten Nations', *Health Affairs*, Summer.

Blendon, R.J., Donelan, K., Jovell, A.J., Pellisé, L., Lombardia, E.C. (1991), 'Spain's Citizens Assess Their Health Care System', *Health Affairs*, Fall.

Evans, R.G. (1981), 'Incomplete Vertical Integration: the Distinctive Structure of the Health Care Industry', in van der Gaag, J. and Perlman, M. (eds), *Health, Economics and Health Economics*, Amsterdam: North-Holland.

Financial Times (1995), 'US employers' health costs fall', February 15, p. 4.

Glennerster, H., Matsaganis, M., Owens, P. and Hancock, S. (1994), 'GP Fundholding: Wild Card or Winning Hand?' in Robinson, R. and Le Grand, J. (eds), *Evaluating the NHS Reforms*, London: King's Fund Institute.

HMSO (1992), *The Health of the Nation*, London: HMSO.

HMSO (1989), *Working for Patients*, London, HMSO.

HMSO (1994), *Managing the New NHS*, London: HMSO.

National Audit Office (1994), *General Practitioner Fundholding in England*, London: HMSO.

Organization for Economic Cooperation and Development (1992), *The Reform of Health Care: A Comparative Analysis of Seven OECD Countries*, Paris: OECD.

Organization for Economic Cooperation and Development (1993), *Health Systems, Facts and Trends*, Paris: OECD.

Organization for Economic Cooperation and Development (1994), *The Reform of Health Care Systems: A Review of Seventeen OECD Countries*, Paris: OECD.

Royal College of General Practitioners (1992), *The European Study of Referrals from Primary to Secondary Care*, Occasional Paper 56, April.

Social and Community Planning Research (1994), *British Social Attitudes Survey*, 8th Report

Social and Community Planning Research (1994) *British Social Attitudes Survey*, 11th Report.

Schieber G.J., Poullier, J.P. and Greenwald, M. (1991), 'Health Care Systems in Twenty-Four Countries', *Health Affairs*, Fall.

The White House (1993), *Health Security, Preliminary Plan Summary*, Washington DC.

3 Health, hierarchy and hominids – biological correlates of the socioeconomic gradient in health*

Robert G. Evans

Political epidemiology: social inequalities in health

Top People live longer, and they are healthier while doing so. Fifteen years after the pioneering work of the Black Report (Townsend and Davidson 1988), nearly twenty years after the observations of growing health inequalities that led to the appointment of the Research Working Group, the correlation of health with social status is now so extensively documented and so widely recognized that it has even come to the attention of *The Economist* (1994a). The efforts by the UK government in 1980 to suppress the Black Report, presumably in the hope that its findings would go away, have been spectacularly unsuccessful. The study of health inequalities is now a significant research sub-industry; and socioeconomic gradients have turned up in every country where researchers have looked for them.

Although the existence of the correlation is no longer in question, the interpretation remains highly contentious. *Why* are class differences so strongly correlated with the prevalence of disease and the risk of death, and what, if anything, can or should be done about it? Interpretation has from the very beginning been tightly entangled with political ideology and economic interest.

The logical sequence from observation, to explanation, to response, is often turned on its head. Conflicting views of what constitutes a well-ordered society (depending in large part on one's position in that society) determine preferences for particular social policies, and these in turn influence the choice of explanations.

For those on the Left, health inequalities are clear evidence of material deprivation, symptoms of an unjust society.[1] Only by a more equitable distribution of both life chances and rewards can one hope to improve the health of the least healthy, and this in turn is the key to improving the overall health of

---

*This paper draws heavily on work by the members of the Program in Population Health, Canadian Institute for Advanced Research, which is presented in more detail in R.G. Evans, M.L. Barer and T.R. Marmor (eds), *Why Are Some People Healthy and Others Not? The Determinants of Health of Populations*, New York: Aldine de Gruyter, 1994.

the population. To become healthier, we must remake our societies. Among other things, this will require a significant redistribution of wealth and power from the more to the less fortunate. The improvement of health, for which there is widespread public support, can thus be recruited to advance a broader and more contentious social agenda.

To those on the Right, however, this looks like a fool's errand. The first knee-jerk reaction is that the correlation is spurious, that health status determines social position rather than the other way around. Fitter, healthier people rise in a just society that rewards performance. As to *why* they are fitter – perhaps because of genetic superiority or early life experience – well, that is just the way life is. And anyway, people lower down the social scale actually *choose* their unhealthy circumstances. They smoke, eat bad diets, do not get enough exercise, and in general fail to look after themselves. (This is clearly the explanation favoured by *The Economist*.) If they are sicker, and die sooner, it is their own fault. Medical care is provided at public expense; but there is not much more that can, or in any case should, be done, except perhaps to lecture the badly behaved about 'taking more responsibility for their own health'.

Each of these lines of interpretation has significant problems of fact and logic, and in both political preferences for particular remedies – income redistribution, or *laissez-faire* – clearly influence the favoured perceptions of mechanism. But the debate has already generated a large literature and a further critique in this paper would add little. Moreover it is difficult to enter the discussion without simultaneously becoming involved in the political controversy that must inevitably surround claims of 'inequalities' – particularly inequalities with mortal consequences. Instead I shall try to reframe the discussion of class and health in a way which may hold the political and ideological issues at arm's length, at least for a time, while also broadening the range of relevant evidence.

Heterogeneities in health: moral offence or research opportunity
Socioeconomic status (SES) is only one among any number of measures by which to partition a population, and not an unambiguous one at that. The British are commonly regarded as suffering from a morbid fascination with social class, giving it the sort of attention that in other countries would be reserved for sex, or federal–provincial fiscal relations. Elsewhere it is less clear what 'class' means, or how it should be identified, perhaps using measures of income, education, occupational status or public esteem.

In practice people are grouped on the basis of some measurable indicator variable or variables which are accepted as standing for the more abstract notion of SES. (In the US a key indicator seems to be race.) But one could equally well categorize a population by region, or sex, or ethnic status, or religious affiliation, or height, and so on. If one found systematic differences in health between the sub-populations thus defined, one could then refer to 'health inequalities' across these divides as well. Such language, however, automatically combines an observation of differentness with an implicit judgement of unfairness that may or may not be appropriate. It is well known, for example, that women in industrialized societies live, on average, significantly longer than men. But this 'health inequality' generates little or no political controversy; to my knowledge no government has ever tried to suppress the evidence.

A more neutral term, *heterogeneities*, captures the generic observation that when populations are partitioned by some variable of interest, significant health differences are frequently found between the groups (Hertzman et al. 1994). Comparing these sub-populations may then provide clues to determine the causal factors in differences in health, without simultaneously implying (or denying) that these differences represent 'inequalities' in the sense of indicators of injustice. Inequalities are goads to action; heterogeneities are merely guides to research. '...[T]here is a tremendous potential to exploit heterogeneity in populations as a wedge for greater understanding' (Sapolsky 1993).

Such greater understanding, once achieved, may indeed have significant moral or political implications. But the more neutral language is less likely to trigger ideological immune systems at the very beginning of the process.

A focus on heterogeneities as 'a wedge for greater understanding' then leads us to consider *mechanisms* rather than remedies. What are the pathways through which some groups of people become healthier than others? Material deprivation is certainly one possible explanation, and has the attraction that the links between deprivation and ill-health – hunger, exposure, crowding, environmental toxins – are relatively easy to imagine. But so are the 'self-abuse' explanations of the Right – smoking, overeating, too much television.

Political debates select the simple, easily communicated explanation, which is usually seriously incomplete if not outright wrong. In reality the pathways through which heterogeneities in health status emerge seem to be a good deal more complex than is contemplated, or caricatured, by either side. But the quick, easily understood, politically comfortable 'explanations', with their associated prepackaged policy remedies, tend to crowd out the messages that are emerging from more wide-ranging and subtle efforts to understand the relation between status and health.

The third step in seeking a more neutral stance is to broaden our interests from heterogeneities in *human* populations to include consideration of other primates closely related to ourselves. The old-world monkeys are particularly well adapted for these comparisons. Apart from genetic and physiological similarities, they have complex and sophisticated social structures with readily identifiable status hierarchies. There are several long-term research programmes studying different species, some in the wild and some under experimental conditions, that have generated findings remarkably consistent with those emerging from observations in the human species.

This paper will draw particularly heavily on findings from two remarkable programmes of research with free-living primate populations. Both populations have a well-defined hierarchical structure, and in both one finds strong connections between this hierarchy and factors related to health. The research design and procedures are, however, very different and are in important ways complementary. When taken together each study provides important insights that are missing from the other, because interventions and modes of data collection that are impossible in one are possible in the other.

Robert Sapolsky has for fourteen years been studying a population of wild baboons in the Serengeti ecosystem of East Africa, and has assembled a remarkable array of information on the relationship between physiology and social structure. For an even longer period Michael Marmot has been studying the experiences of a group of over 10,000 British civil servants in the Whitehall ecosystem of London.

Hierarchy and health among the hominids of Whitehall
Perhaps the clearest message to emerge from the first decade of the Whitehall studies was that there is a correlation between status and mortality, and it is *large*. Figure 3.1, which has been widely reproduced, shows that when (male) individuals were followed over a ten-year period, those in the lowest civil service grades had three times as large a probability (age-adjusted) of dying as those at the top. More recent work has shown that this gradient has persisted through the 1980s, and is observed for measures of illness as well as death, and for females as well as males (Marmot et al. 1991; North et al. 1993).

These observations are of particular importance because they are *person-specific* as well as *population-based*. They are drawn from the experience of a large population of identified individuals, followed through time. Other studies correlating mortality and SES, and particularly the data from the British Office of Population Censuses and Surveys (OPCS) which were drawn upon in the Black Report, have been subjected to a number of methodological criticisms. Some have been based on aggregate data, comparing averages among groups that were not always strictly comparable, rather than following the experience of actual individuals. Their messages are powerfully confirmed by the Whitehall findings.[2]

Marmot's work, however, also highlighted two other features of the relationship between hierarchy and health which deserve special attention. The first is that it is a *gradient* and not a threshold, and the second is that it is observed for most (though not all) causes of death.

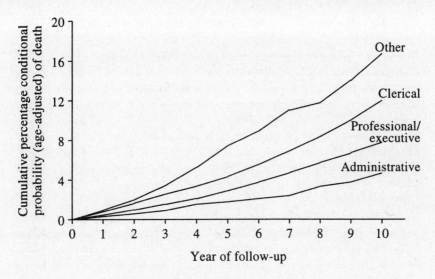

*Figure 3.1   Whitehall study: all-cause mortality among total population by
year of follow-up*

As shown in Figure 3.1, the mortality curves improve steadily as one
moves up the hierarchy. Death rates are lower in the top administrative grades
than in the professional and executive grades just below them. But people in
the latter can hardly be described as living in destitution. Indeed all those in
the study are employed, and in jobs which do not expose them to the same
occupational hazards as, say, lumbering or fishing. Material deprivation cannot explain the observations in Figure 3.1. This is not to say that deprivation
does not exist, or that it is not harmful to health. But there is clearly a process
at work by which hierarchy influences health status directly, independently of
deprivation.

The understanding of this gradient in health status is not assisted, therefore, by the automatic assumption that it is a problem of 'the poor', those
folks over there, who are to be cherished or spurned according to one's
political predilections but are, in any case, 'other'. There is more to health
inequality than poverty; *de te fabula narratur*, this story is about us.

Furthermore, in the modern world people are required to die *of* something.
('Visitation of God' is no longer fashionable on death certificates.) Aggregate
mortality differentials should be reflected in differentials in causes of death
from particular diseases, and (as shown in Table 3.1) they are. What is
interesting is that there are gradients in mortality rates for almost all diseases.
There is no preferred channel of effect. This suggests that hierarchical position may be associated with some sort of underlying vulnerability or vitality,

Table 3.1   Age-adjusted relative mortality in ten years by civil service
grade and cause of death*

Cause of death	Administrative	Professional & executive	Clerical	Other
Lung cancer	0.5	1.0	2.2	3.6
Other cancer	0.8	1.0	1.4	1.4
Coronary heart disease	0.5	1.0	1.4	1.7
Cerebro-vascular disease	0.3	1.0	1.4	1.2
Chronic bronchitis	0.0	1.0	6.0	7.3
Other respiratory	1.1	1.0	2.6	3.1
Gastro-intestinal diseases	0.0	1.0	1.6	2.8
Genito-urinary diseases	1.3	1.0	0.7	3.1
Accidents and homicide	0.0	1.0	1.4	1.5
Suicide	0.7	1.0	1.0	1.9
Non-smoking-related causes				
Cancer	0.8	1.0	1.3	1.4
Non-cancer	0.6	1.0	1.5	2.0
All causes	0.6	1.0	1.6	2.1

*   Calculated from logistic equation adjusting for age.

Source: Marmot (1986) p. 25

that is expressed through a number of different diseases. The diseases themselves are not the critical mechanisms.

Of particular importance, the gradients are found for both the smoking-
and non-smoking-related diseases (Tables 3.1 and 3.2). As everyone knows,
the lower classes smoke and the middle and upper classes do not. Smoking
causes lung cancer, emphysema, and bronchitis, and is a risk factor for many
other diseases, especially heart disease – tobacco is an addictive, toxic substance. So they bring it on themselves – what can one do? Well, before
throwing one's hands in the air, one might at least wonder *why* smoking is
now so clearly socially graded, in all our societies. If it were simply a 'taste',
or even a genetic predisposition to addiction, one would expect smoking
behaviour to be spread more equally across the population, not concentrated

Table 3.2   Age-adjusted mortality in ten years (and number of deaths from coronary heart disease and lung cancer) by grade and smoking status

Cause of death	Administrative	Professional & executive	Clerical	Other	Total
Non-smokers					
CHD	1.40	2.36	2.08	6.89	2.59
Lung cancer	0.00	0.24	0.00	0.25	0.21
Ex-smokers					
CHD	1.29	3.06	3.32	3.98	3.09
Lung cancer	0.21	0.59	0.56	1.05	0.62
Current smokers					
CHD	2.16	3.58	4.92	6.62	4.00
Lung cancer	0.35	0.73	1.49	2.33	2.00

CHD: Coronary heart disease

Source: Marmot (1986) p. 26.

at the low end. But that is a separate issue. The main point is that the Whitehall gradient is not explained by differences in smoking behaviour.

The correlates of cardiovascular disease, which is the largest single cause of death, have been extensively explored. Marmot and his colleagues (1978) have partitioned the gradient in cardiac mortality according to the differences in the three individual characteristics – smoking, hypertension, and blood lipid levels – which are most widely accepted as risk factors. The results are shown in Figure 3.2. These factors *do* explain a portion of the difference in death rates between those at the top and those at the bottom of the hierarchy, but what is most apparent is how much they leave unexplained. Something else, something important, is at work.

This large hierarchical gradient in mortality, not apparently linked to material deprivation, and expressed through a number of different causes of death, also emerges in the longitudinal data from the OPCS that were used in the Black Report. Differential mortality by social class can be found, as shown in Table 3.3, at least back to 1911. But the principal causes of death have changed radically over that period, implying that the factor or factors underlying the gradient have been independent of the diseases themselves. What-

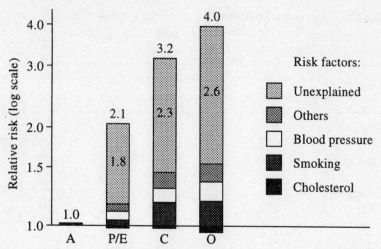

A: Administrative;   P/E Professional/Executive;   C: Clerical;   O: Other

Source: Marmot et al. (1978) p. 248.

Figure 3.2   Relative risk of CHD death in different grades 'explained' by risk factors (age-standardized)

ever diseases are the chief killers, people lower down in the hierarchy are always more at risk.

The historical data also span a period of remarkable expansion in the medical care services – expansions in scale and capacity, technical sophistication and access. Whatever criticisms one may make of health care systems in the UK or anywhere else, it is undeniable that over the last century and particularly over the last half-century their reach has been extended as never before. While it would be naive to claim that class differences in access have disappeared as a result, access has at least become a great deal less unequal. And without accepting the more extreme claims of the medical miracle marketeers, there is obvious evidence of improved effectiveness in cure, care, and contribution in quality of life. Yet the social gradient, in the UK at least, persists and even grows wider.

Most modern health care is in fact illness care. This is nothing to apologize for; illness care is obviously worth doing, and is often done very well. But if hierarchy influences health in some way more fundamental than the particular illnesses through which differences in health are expressed, then we should not perhaps be surprised if they are unaffected by responses to illness *per se*. Thus the apparent insensitivity of the SES gradient to the massive expansion of the health services, over a period of decades, is not evidence

Table 3.3   *Mortality by social class, 1911–81 (men, 15–64 years, England and Wales)*

Year	Social class				
	Professional	Managerial	Skilled manual and non-manual	Semi-skilled	Unskilled
	I	II	III	IV	V
1911	88	94	96	93	142
1921	82	94	95	101	125
1931	90	94	97	102	111
1951	86	92	101	104	118
1961*	76 (75)	81	100	103	143 (127)
1971*	77 (75)	81	104	114	137 (121)
1981**	66	76	103	116	166

*   To facilitate comparisons, figures shown in parentheses have been adjusted to the classification of occupations used in 1951.
**   Men, 20–64 years, UK.
Note: Figures are SMRs, which express age-adjusted mortality rates as a percentage of the national average at each date.

Source: Wilkinson (1986) p. 2 and Office of Population Censuses and Surveys (1978) p. 174.

that those services are not doing their job. But it is at least suggestive that there is something else going on that may be beyond their reach.

The historical persistence of the SES gradient in the OPCS data also supports the Whitehall studies, in undercutting explanations based on material deprivation. The present economic environment, with slow growth and a growing disparity of incomes between rich and poor, raises the possibility of an absolute decline in living standards for those low down the social scale. It is tempting to correlate this with the growing disparities in health status. Over the century as a whole, however, absolute living standards have obviously risen a great deal, even for those at the bottom. It should then be clear from the historical record that the declining prevalence of deprivation, in absolute terms, leads to declining health inequalities. But as shown in Table 3.3, it does not.

Again it should be emphasized that this is *not* to imply the irrelevance of material conditions. *The World Development Report 1993*, issued by the World Bank (1993), provides a dramatic comparison across countries of the relation between average incomes and mortality (Figure 3.4; see also Preston 1976, p. 67). At the lowest income levels the relation between mortality and

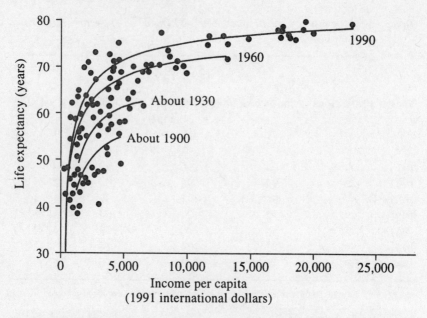

Note: International dollars are derived from national currencies not by use of exchange rates but by assessment of purchasing power. The effect is to raise the relative incomes of poorer countries, often substatially.

Source: World Bank (1993), p. 34.

Figure 3.3   Life expectancy and income per capita for selected countries and periods

income is very clear. But over time an increasing number of countries are reaching a plateau where more income does not appear to be correlated with further reductions in mortality.[3]

Within a single country, greater affluence can contribute through a number of channels to better health. But the fact that the *gradient* in mortality in the UK has not been reduced, even during times when living standards were improving across the whole population, weakens any explanation in terms of absolute deprivation. Wilkinson (1992) considers the UK experience in the context of several different sets of data on income and mortality in developed societies. These suggest quite strongly that life expectancy is correlated, not with the level of income *per se*, but with how equally it is distributed. This in turn implies that it is relative, not absolute, income that matters within each country.

So we are led to think about factors or processes associated with hierarchy, which can exert a powerful influence on health status independent of material conditions, or even of 'lifestyles' as traditionally represented, expressed through a number of different diseases. At this point, we shift our attention to the second major study of free-ranging primates, that of the Kenyan olive baboons.

Health and hierarchy among the cercopithecids of Kenya

Sapolsky's studies begin from an interest in endocrinology and stress physiology, and the growing body of evidence indicating that people's physiological responses to stress are profoundly influenced by their emotional make-up, their personalities, and their positions in society (Sapolsky 1990). Ideally, to understand these relationships would require simultaneous observation of the structure and interactions of an entire social group, and various physiological measures of its members.

But there are severe restrictions, both ethical and practical, on what is possible in the study of human populations. Many of the interesting interactions – mating, grooming, feeding, confrontation and conflict – take place under cover, not on the open plain. Even if one could follow an individual continuously, one would miss most of the group action. Moreover, Sapolsky's basic technique consists of anaesthetic darting of subjects, as unobtrusively as possible, so as to take physiological measures in particular circumstances. It is difficult to imagine a researcher being permitted to dart a senior, or even a middle-level, civil servant during a particularly stressful meeting, in order to measure hormone levels.[4]

On the other hand, caged animals under experimental conditions are already under stress and in artificial environments, and it is hard to know how severe an effect this has on their baseline physiological status and patterns of response.

Free-ranging animals offer a middle ground for research, being more accessible than humans and less 'contaminated' than caged populations. As for the baboons:

> These intelligent animals are good stand-ins for human subjects in part because their primary sources of stress, like those of humans in modern society, are psychological rather than physical. Food is plentiful; the baboons spend only a few hours each day feeding. Predators are few, and infant mortality is low. With the luxury of plentiful resources and free time, the animals can devote themselves to distressing one another. I study the males, who are quite adept at that activity. (Sapolsky 1990)

The individual interactions within the troop are not, however, a simple 'war of all against all', but rather a highly complex social web with a well-defined dominance hierarchy. Status among females tends to be inherited and maintained over the lifetime. But males typically rise in rank as they mature, winning higher positions through overt aggression, holding them through 'threats, psychological harassment, and bluff' (Sapolsky 1993) and then being displaced as their strength declinês with age. The competitive interactions may be individual, but may also involve alliances and combinations – it is good to have friends – which are nonetheless rather unstable.

When the population is divided into dominants and subordinates, the top and bottom halves of the rank order, there are systematic physiological differences between these groups. '…[W]hen the dominance hierarchy is stable (as it usually is), the workings of nearly every physiologic system I have examined differ between the dominant and subordinate males' (Sapolsky 1990). In particular, their endocrine systems function differently in response to stress, as expressed in the 'fight or flight' syndrome.

Like ourselves, or any other animal, the baboons respond to an actual attack or injury or a perceived threat by mobilizing physical and intellectual resources to respond – to fight back or to run away. The neural system interprets the external threat and triggers the release of hormones that direct this process. Maintenance, repair and 'investment' (growth, development and reproduction) are shut down while all available metabolic resources are used to cope with the immediate threat.

But mobilization is expensive. Tissues and organs that are held in a high state of readiness, and denied maintenance and repair, become fatigued and eventually atrophy. The suppression of immune function, which is energy-intensive, puts the individual at greater risk of infection. It is therefore advantageous to be able not only to turn on the 'fight or flight' response rapidly, but also to turn it off when the threat is past. In general, dominant animals are better able to turn off their stress responses.[5]

Subordinate animals appear to be living in a chronic state of stress response, that by analogy with engineering usage we might refer to as chronic strain.[6] The physiological threats come not so much directly from the external environment, but from their own responses to that environment. Recall that most of the stress experienced by these animals is generated by their social interactions rather than by external threats such as predators or lack of food. Moreover most of those stresses are psychological – threats, bluff and harassment rather than outright attack. What really bothers subordinates is not so much being attacked by a leopard, or even worrying about being attacked by a leopard. It is being yawned at by a higher-ranking male (showing very large canine teeth) from a distance of three feet, whenever one is trying to enjoy one's dinner or mate.

The hormonal patterns associated with chronic strain are also associated with a number of different diseases. The suppression of immune system function has already been noted. Sapolsky also finds that the ratio of HDL to LDL, high- to low-density lipoprotein, is lowered in low status males.

Elevated LDL concentrations are risk factors for heart disease in both humans and baboons, and high concentrations of HDL are protective. Moreover there is experimental evidence that sustained glucocorticoid overexposure can suppress HDL:LDL ratios; and basal levels of cortisol, the primate (and human) form of glucocorticoid, are higher in the subordinate baboons.

With proper allowance for scientific caution, what *can* be said is that these studies have demonstrated a *potential* pathway leading from hierarchical position, through differential endocrine responses to stress, to differences in basal hormone levels which are consistent with differential risk status for a number of diseases. These results are in a sense the mirror image of Marmot's findings, where the endpoints are firm – hierarchy correlates unambiguously with mortality – but what is going on between them is much less clear. Working with non-human primates, Sapolsky can characterize in much more detail the physiological characteristics of subjects at different levels in the hierarchy. But the unambiguous connection between status and survival is not so clear.[7]

In neither population is material deprivation a significant part of the story. The dominant primates in both populations get the choicest bits of food, but everyone gets enough to eat. However, the subordinate civil servants also show some physiological signs suggesting chronic strain. Marmot and Theorell (1988) report that both high- and low-ranking civil servants have higher blood pressures when at work than when at home. But while their pressures at work are on average similar, the drop in pressure on going home is significantly greater in the higher-ranking workers.

Hierarchy and health in captive (non-human) primate populations

Experimental studies with captive populations offer more opportunities for intervention. Hamm et al. (1983) showed that feeding a 'moderate' cholesterol diet to cynomolgus macacques will induce heart disease. But when the animals were kept caged in single-sex groups, and their status hierarchies observed, it was found that the degree of occlusion of the coronary arteries in the lowest-status animals in each group was much greater than in the high-status group – twice as high for males, and nearly four times for females.[8] Part of this difference was associated with lower ratios of HDL:LDL in submissive animals – paralleling Sapolsky's findings – and part seemed to be an independent effect.

The degree of occlusion was significantly greater for males than for females: dominant males had about the same degree of occlusion as submissive females (23.1 per cent vs 24 per cent) while submissive males had 44 per cent occlusion, and dominant females only 6.9 per cent. So both diet and gender matter, as they do for humans. But so, independently and significantly, does hierarchical position.

There is a substantial and growing literature, reviewed by Cox (1993), on the relationship between psychosocial factors and immune function in non-human primates. Experimental findings go back nearly thirty years, demonstrating that 'the formation and disruption of social relationships should be viewed as significant psychobiological events with many immunological sequelae, especially for the young monkey'. The endocrine system has traditionally been considered to be the 'mediating pathway', but more recently attention has shifted to the sympathetic nervous system (Cox, 1993, p. 299). Virtually all these findings, however, are under experimental conditions. Sapolsky extends them to free-living conditions, and focuses particularly on the psychosocial consequences of hierarchical position in a way that provides a direct link to the correlations between status and health in hominid populations.

Which comes first, social status or health status?

The obvious question, of course, is that of causality. If dominants and subordinates differ in their endocrine function, as they do, and if this has significant implications for their health, as it might, is this a *consequence* of their differential status, or simply an indicator of differential fitness? Are some 'born to rule'? (This interpretation is quite popular with those of high status in human populations – the cream rises to the top, and the universe unfolds as it should.)

Like all good questions, this one turns out not to have a simple answer – or rather, the simple answer is 'Yes and No'.

The stress of social circumstances induces physiological responses

In the first place, the subordinate baboons' greater difficulty in regulating their basal cortisol levels, in turning off the 'fight or flight' response, seems to be induced rather than innate. Experiments in other animals (including humans) have shown that '[p]rolonged or repeated stressors will elevate basal glucocorticoid concentrations and cause feedback resistance…'. This mechanism may also be at work in the subordinate baboons, such that the stressfulness of their social status leads, through frequent triggering of the fight or flight response, to blunting of feedback sensitivity and permanently elevated basal cortisol levels.

Consistent with this, observations of dominant males during periods in which the status hierarchy is disrupted and status is uncertain, show that they have the high basal cortisol levels and physiological response patterns characteristic of subordinates. Even though they remain dominant as a group, the uncertainty of their individual status leads to reduced efficiency of endocrine function, and symptoms of chronic strain. '[T]he optimal hormonal profile seen in dominant males during stable times is an effect and not a cause of one's high rank' (Sapolsky 1990, p. 121).

Again these findings can be reinforced from the study of captive populations under experimental conditions. A number of studies of dominant males in unstable captive social groups, (cited in Sapolsky 1993, p. 459) have found that dominant males do not have the low basal cortisol levels typically observed during more peaceful times.

Cohen et al. (1992) demonstrated a direct link between instability and vulnerability. They randomly assigned male cynomolgus macacques to 'stable' and 'unstable' living conditions, and followed them over a 26-month period. The animals were housed in groups of four or five, and for half the population, these groups remained the same throughout the study. But for the other half, the housing groups were 'shuffled' every month. The animals had repeatedly to adapt to living with a new set of companions. At the end of the period, it was found that their immune responses were significantly depressed, relative to those who had been living in stable social conditions.

The endocrinal differences among the baboons were directly linked to the frequency and outcomes of 'personal' confrontations. Dominant animals that were being challenged from below, and whose status was in question, showed chronic strain patterns even though they might still be winning the majority of their confrontations. On the other hand, frequent confrontations with those of *higher* rank, and occasional reversals of status, do not seem to lead to chronic strain – moving up is good for you.

In one particular instance, however, a male changed troops and adopted a strategy of aggressively 'going for dominance' in the new troop. This significantly increased the overall hormonal evidence of strain in the members of the new troop. But *individuals* in that troop showed greater or lesser responses, according to the frequency of their interactions with the newcomer. Of particular importance, the highest cortisol concentrations and lowest lymphocyte counts in the troop were shown by the newcomer himself. The highly aggressive strategy was costly in physiological terms. Far from being 'born to rule', the newcomer was engaged in a very stressful gamble that, if successful, would put him in a position to relax and enjoy the benefits, endocrinal and otherwise, of rank.

There is thus clear evidence that hierarchical status influences physiology, in ways that could influence vulnerability to a whole range of diseases. But the linkage from status to sickness is not simple, direct, or complete. The physical effects on the individual depend upon how that status is experienced. Dominance that is stable, and maintained by the occasional reminder of showing one's large teeth, is much more restful than dominance that is under constant challenge, with uncertain outcomes.

Subordination, however, implies (among other things) being the recipient of 'displaced aggression' – being attacked out of the blue by a higher-ranking male who has lost a confrontation higher up the line. But the frequency of these events varies from group to group and year to year; there are definitely better and worse times and places to be a subordinate.

The place of innate 'personality'

The powerful evidence of the importance of social environment, however, does not rule out a role for individual characteristics as well. While hormonal function is related to rank, it is also clearly related to what can only be described as 'personality'. The 'optimal hormonal profile' is found only in some of the dominant animals; others are much more similar to subordinates. And there is a well-defined set of personality traits and behaviours associated with this profile. They include ability to read social situations accurately, to distinguish real threats from behavioural 'noise', and to respond actively and successfully to such threats. If unsuccessful, 'displace your aggression' – if you lose a confrontation or a fight, get it out of your system by beating up someone else.

But 'true dominants' also spend more time playing with infants, and are more likely to have female 'friends' as distinct from mates; they spend more time grooming and being groomed by non-estrus females. (Rates of sexual contacts, however, as opposed to affiliative ones, were not associated with cortisol levels.) Baboons with this more 'laid-back' personality spent a longer time in the dominant cohort of the troop – recall that dominance in males is not permanent but rather gained and lost over the life cycle. But this style is not a learned behaviour: 'the lower basal cortisol trait is present in the very first season of such males' long tenures; it is a predictor, rather than a consequence of such social success' (Sapolsky 1993, p. 465).

Again the captive studies offer supporting evidence. Cohen et al., comparing macaques in 'stable' and 'unstable' social settings, found that various forms of 'affiliative behaviour' were more common in the unstable environments, and that the animals engaging in such behaviour showed far less depression of immune function. Those able to increase their affiliative behaviours were largely protected against the effects of social instability. Some are better than others at making friends and, in an unstable environment, this can be good for your health.

Sapolsky (1993, pp. 465–6) provides a particularly apt summary:

> although social rank is an important predictor of some physiological parameters, just as important can be the type of society in which that rank occurs, and the way in which one experiences such a rank...[moreover]...the filters of personality with which an individual views these events and the varying strategies available for coping with them are probably immensely important variables as well.

Coming back to the hominids, research shows that 'in the face of overt and undeniable external stressors, the magnitude of the physiological stress response can be modulated enormously by psychological factors...by increasing the individual's sense of control, of predictability, by providing outlets for frustration, and by strengthening social support networks'.

Is biology – or sociology – destiny?

The importance of 'personality' leaves open the question of malleability. To what extent are people, or baboons, born with protective or vulnerable personalities, as part of their genetic make-up? How much of personality is acquired through life experience, and how? Can 'coping styles' be modified to decrease vulnerability to 'the stress of life'?

There is a related question of malleability at the societal level. All human societies have hierarchies. Are their effects on health therefore inevitable, simply a part of the human condition, or are the individual experiences of dominance or subordination, and the corresponding physiological effects, quite as variable among hominids as they appear to be among baboons?

Some hierarchies are rougher than others

The second question seems easier to answer, at least in part. Vågerö and Lundberg (1989) have categorized the Swedish population by the same social class measures as used in the UK by the OPCS and presented in the Black Report, and have calculated the corresponding class-specific mortality rates. A gradient emerges even in egalitarian Sweden, with higher age-standardized mortality (for middle-aged males) as one goes down the class ladder. But the difference from top to bottom is much smaller in Sweden, and the mortality rates among the lowest class of Swedes is lower than among the highest class in the UK.

Kunst and Mackenbach (1992) have studied mortality gradients among men in several countries in Western Europe, using both education and occupational status as measures of SES. All countries show status gradients, but the slope of the gradient is much greater in some than in others. Moreover the countries themselves show a consistent ranking in their slopes. The gradients tend to be flattest in Denmark and the Netherlands, growing larger as one moves to Norway and Sweden, then to Finland and England and Wales, larger again in the US, with France and Italy having the steepest gradients of all.

As they point out, gradients in mortality depend on both the degree of inequality in the underlying measure and the extent to which these inequalities are translated into health differences. A steep mortality gradient could be observed either because of large inequalities on the SES measure used, or because such inequalities as exist have a relatively large impact on mortality (or both). Kunst and Mackenbach conclude that the former is true of the US, and the latter of France and Italy.

The implication seems to be that gradients in health status are *not* an inevitable part of the human condition – at least not on the scale which we now observe. Societies can be organized in ways which accentuate or buffer the effects which give rise to those gradients – that seems to be beyond debate. But there is still ample room for controversy over what exactly are the critical features of different societies that determine the slope of these gradients, not only because our knowledge is incomplete, but because here we come back to the inherent conflicts of interest between people at different levels in the hierarchy.

It may be worth emphasizing, however, that the baboon studies do not show that you have to remake the society from top to bottom in order to mitigate the health effects of hierarchy. It may be enough to reduce the extent to which those of lower status have their faces rubbed in it. What seems to be physiologically harmful is the chronic strain, the elevated cortisol level and other elements of a 'sub-optimal hormonal profile' that come from being subjected to frequent and unpredictable attack, both physical and particularly psychological.

Genetics matters – but is not predestination
The malleability of the individual, even in principle, is, however, a more complex question. Could one identify and inculcate 'coping styles' and personality traits that leave people less vulnerable to external stress? Or are these genetically predetermined?

Studies of other primates again suggest part of the answer. Working with rhesus monkeys, Suomi (1991) finds that about 20 per cent of the population have 'reactive' personalities such that they experience extreme behavioural and physiological responses to external stresses (see also Cox 1993, p. 301). There are certain stages in the animal's life that are periods of high stress – separation from the mother when she resumes breeding, or (for males) expulsion from the natal troop. The behavioural responses to these stresses by highly reactive animals differ, at different stages of the life cycle: 'teenagers' behave differently from infants, but the underlying physiological patterns are the same. Extreme reactions to stress can put at risk the health and even the survival of the animal.

Suomi and his colleagues have shown that this pattern of reactivity is inherited; they have even been able to breed for reactivity. This suggests that 'coping styles' for dealing with stress may also be inherited in the baboon, or the human.[9] But they also found that reactive infants that received particularly competent nurturing, from their own or from foster mothers, did not display the extreme physiological and behavioural responses to stress and indeed might be more capable as adults. Conversely several studies reviewed by Cox (1993) found that disruption of normal rearing conditions very early in the life of young monkeys led to long-term reductions in their immune competence.

There seems little support for the proposition that human social classes, however defined, represent genetically distinct populations. A more promising line of argument generalizes from Suomi's observation that genetic vulnerability can be socially buffered. Geneticists increasingly emphasize the interplay between genetic predisposition and environment, as opposed to older notions of genetic determinism (e.g. Baird, 1994). Whether or not a genetic predisposition will in fact be expressed depends upon the experiences of the individual organism, particularly in early life. Genetic advantages and disadvantages may be equally distributed across the population, but the environmental resources necessary to compensate for disadvantages (or to exploit advantages) are not.

The biological 'embeddedness' of early experience

This perspective finds support in the Kauai longitudinal study of the 1955 birth cohort from that island (Werner 1989a). One of the findings has been that children who suffer moderate or severe perinatal stress, but are reared in 'good' environments (as measured by family stability or high socioeconomic status) suffer little or no disadvantage in development at 20 months. Children in unstable households but with no perinatal stress, likewise showed little disadvantage. But perinatal stress *plus* poor rearing environment had quite severe consequences for child development.

Studies of the effects of childhood exposure to lead on intellectual development show a strikingly similar pattern. In general, the more exposure, the more impairment. Severe exposure impairs intelligence severely, regardless of the quality of the rearing environment. But for children with 'moderate' exposure, the degree of impairment is much less if the rearing environment is of high quality (Bellinger et al. 1993).

The Kauai and lead studies do not address the issue of genetic endowment versus environment, but they do show that superior rearing environments can compensate for the effects of adverse exposures at or shortly after birth. They parallel, 'in the human', the non-human primate studies showing that the early rearing experience can have long-term effects on physiological functioning. The impact of the early psychosocial environment thus seems to be just as 'real' as that of the physicochemical environment, with a similar potential for becoming permanently embedded in the biology of the individual.

One of the best-known findings of the Kauai study has been the identification of a small group of 'vulnerable but invincible' or 'indomitable' children who despite 'high risk' perinatal experiences and home environments grew into successful adults (Werner and Smith 1982; Werner 1989b). The common characteristics seemed to be close bonding with and high level of attention from *some* adult – not necessarily a parent or even a family member – very early in life. But these children also had cheerful, outgoing personalities that 'elicit positive responses', presumably enabling them to recruit emotional support, and again emphasizing that the question 'nature *or* nurture?' is profoundly misleading.

By their early 30s, however, these 'vulnerable but invincible' people were showing a significantly higher proportion of self-reported health problems, of a sort consistent with stress (Werner 1989b). One is reminded of Sapolsky's observation of the baboon who changed troops and made a very aggressive bid for status; his hormonal profile suggested the highest level of strain in the troop. Compensation may have a biological price.

The determinants of health and the sources of the SES gradient
The emerging evidence on the determinants of health, coming from a wide range of disciplines, is surveyed in detail in Evans et al. (1994). The introduction to that volume offers an engineering example as a metaphorical summary. The strength of a beam under a load – an external stress – will depend upon what the beam is made of, how it has been made, and how it is supported. The load-bearing characteristics of steel differ from those of wood or glass, but each can be shaped and treated during fabrication in ways which dramatically change performance. And a beam with several supports distributed along its length will carry much more weight before distortion or failure than one that is fastened at one end only, and then extended into space. Metaphorically, we could refer to the beam's genetic endowment, the quality of its early-life rearing, and the supportiveness of its current social environment.

Obviously humans do differ in their genetic endowment. The primate studies strongly suggest that these differences make some people much more vulnerable to being 'bent out of shape' by stress, but that this vulnerability can be compensated by high-quality early life rearing, or increased by poor-quality nurturing. Whether or not vulnerability becomes translated into illness then depends upon the physical and social environment in which the individual finds himself, or herself. Furthermore, the human life course tends to be a good deal more complex than that of most other animals, even our near relatives. Present vulnerability or resilience will depend upon the accumulation of experiences all along the way, but the very early life period appears to be particularly critical for us as well as our relatives (Hertzman 1994).

The resulting variation in individual experiences could then aggregate into the observed correlation between socioeconomic class and health, but not because there are differences in *genetic* make-up between classes. Rather, those higher up in a hierarchy are less exposed to the sorts of psychosocial stresses that induce the endocrinal and neural responses that constitute chronic strain, and lead to a number of forms of physiological damage. They also have more resources, social and economic, with which to respond. Moreover, in so far as higher status among humans tends to be inherited, those of higher rank may on average receive higher-quality early nurturing, and a higher proportion of positive than of negative experiences thereafter, and thus be less vulnerable to, and better able to cope with, whatever stresses they do face. They can carry more stress, with less strain.[10]

Such a general explanation still leaves room for the tough and resilient individual from a deprived background, or the fragile child of privilege. Status, however measured, is a determinant of health only in a statistical sense; good (and bad) genes and nurturing may be found all across the social spectrum. Nor does it rule out the confounding effects of social mobility: robust and healthy individuals *are* more likely to move up, and the sickly to move down. But the non-human primate studies, in which this is *exactly* how status is gained and lost, support the conclusions from studies of human populations, that this cannot be more than a partial explanation for the SES–health link, and that there is a very obvious causal arrow from status to physiological functioning.

The study of non-human primate populations tells us a good deal about the biological processes that link hierarchy with health, and fills in some of the gaps that are inevitably left by studies in human populations. Observations to the effect that the psychosocial environment becomes embedded in the biology of the individual, and that that environment is principally made up of relations with other individuals, seem to generalize fairly smoothly from one primate population to another.

But the precise environmental characteristics that influence health need not be the same in different species. Human and non-human infants probably have similar needs for maternal contact, but different requirements for vocalization: only the humans learn to speak. And it is doubtful if removing the canine teeth of adult males would greatly influence the hierarchical structure of the UK civil service. Thus one should not expect a collection of detailed policy prescriptions for modifying the human social environment to emerge from comparative primatology.

The simple-minded explanations of the Left and Right, with all their faults, lead fairly directly to proposals for action (or inaction). The more complex interplay of genetic predisposition, early-life experience, current stress exposures, and 'learned' or biologically embedded physiological and behavioural response patterns, leaves us with equally complex questions as to appropriate interventions. Nevertheless, some generalizations seem at this point to be defensible.

Health and income: share the wealth, or go for growth?

For most people in affluent societies, there is no simple mechanical linkage
between health and income (Wilkinson 1992). The health gradient appears to
be a consequence, not of material deprivation – 'cold, dampness, filth, mal-
nutrition and starvation, overcrowding and endemic infectious diseases'
(Charlton 1994)[11] – but of patterns of interpersonal relations within a hierarchy. All the primates in the studies above, human and non-human, captive
or free-living, were adequately fed and housed; the stresses they faced were
generated by their fellows. The resulting physiological strains they displayed
depended both on the extent of these stresses, and on their own personal
interpretations and reactions.

But if material deprivation does not explain the health gradient, then
there is no reason why making everybody richer should *in itself* eliminate
it, or raise the average level of health in the group. There *are* very impoverished populations in which absolute deprivation is an important determinant of health, and there are people even in affluent societies whose absolute standard of living places their health at risk. But for most of us income
appears not to be a determinant of health in a functional sense, but rather a
marker (one of many) both for exposure to stress and for the availability of
coping resources and other mechanisms for buffering its physiological effects.

The absence of a simple functional relationship between health and wealth
is not, however, the end of the story. It is not hierarchy *per se*, but the way in
which status is *experienced* by the members of the hierarchy, that affects their
physiological and behavioural responses. There would seem to be at least two
channels through which the overall wealth of a society might influence the
health of its members, and moderate the social gradient, quite independently
of any form of absolute deprivation.

First, affluent societies maintain institutions to protect their members against
external threats, supplementing the resources of individuals and families.
Such collective buffering mechanisms are costly, and inevitably require some
degree of redistribution of resources. But they also affect the extent to which
participation in the society is dependent upon status, as expressed in income
or otherwise.

Of course the rich have bigger cars, but is there also decent public trans-
portation? Of course the rich can enjoy more expensive vacations, but does
everyone have the same access to the same quality of medical care? What
about the educational system – do the bright and hard-working from every
stratum have equal chances? As among the non-human primates, some are
always bigger, stronger, and more aggressive than others, but how often and
how severely do the subordinates get their faces rubbed in that fact? It seems
to make a difference.

A second potential channel of influence has to do with the perception of progress. Economic growth, even if it lifts all the boats together, gives each individual the sense of progress and of hope. Tomorrow will be better than today. This seems to be an important component of psychological well-being, which also translates into physical well-being.

Economic decline both darkens the perceived future of each individual, and erodes collective support for the social mechanisms that buffer stress. If the future is not going to be better than the past for *all* of us, then I want to be sure that I'm all right (Jack). And if that requires pushing you down, too bad.[12] It is no accident that the attack on the welfare state has coincided with the decline in economic growth rates throughout the Western world.

Health care services: part of the solution, and of the problem

Health care in the modern world is largely illness care. In so far as differences in status lead to differences in illness rates, the health services have to deal with the consequences of the gradient. But it is unlikely that they can do much to change it – in any case they do not appear to have done so up to now.[13] One might use differences in SES as a basis for allocating care services across a population, but only as a proxy for differences in needs for care, which it would be preferable to be able to measure directly, not with any expectation that such services would in themselves change the underlying processes at work.

Yet observed health gradients are large, relative to the effects of specific illnesses that the care services do respond to. Flattening the social gradient in mortality, by raising the life expectancy of those at the bottom towards those at the top, could have a greater impact on overall longevity than the complete elimination of a major disease such as cancer. We do not know how to do so; but then we do not know how to eliminate cancer either. Nevertheless massive resources are devoted to biomedical research; the Americans alone have spent $25 billion or so on a self-declared 'War on Cancer' that is now charitably described as 'not won' (Beardsley 1994). Since the social gradient in health is increasingly being provided with a respectable biological basis to link together what have previously been strong but ill-understood correlations, it might repay investigation on the same scale as the more traditional biomedical sciences.

Indeed, the study of the sources of heterogeneity in health status raises some distinctly worrying questions about current trends in the health services, particularly about the futuristic technological fantasies of the Buck Rogers set (*The Economist* 1994b). It is well understood, since the work of McKeown (1979), that medical technology can take much less credit for past improvements in health status than its celebrators have claimed.[14] But this common knowledge does not extend to the general public, or their political representatives. The popular will to believe in miracles is as strong as ever, and the technology marketeers take full advantage.

The steady increases in care costs, against which all developed countries have been struggling with varying success over the last 20 years, are largely a consequence of the ever more intensive servicing of increasingly elderly patients with increasingly sophisticated techniques. All our systems are spending a larger share of their resources treating the elderly, not because there are more of them (the usual claim), but because more and more is being done to each.

But age increases vulnerability to the hormonal changes associated with stress. Animal studies show that, among other things, elevated cortisol levels actually kill off neurons. Worse, they seem to target the very neurons involved in coping with stress (Sapolsky 1992). These studies thus provide biological support for the clinical impression that placing very elderly people in institutions, even for acute care, may render them incapable of independent living thereafter. If 'first do no harm' is to guide medical interventions, the potential for permanent harm from the stress of the intervention itself must be taken into account along with all the other, better-known ways in which too much, or the wrong sort, of care can lead to iatrogenic illness (Stoddart and Lavis 1994).

At the society-wide level, there is still much controversy among economists over the proposition that an overextended health care system may actually weaken a nation's economy and reduce its rate of economic growth. Simple stories about fringe benefit costs and threats to international competitiveness seem easy to refute; the linkages through savings and investment rates and participation in technological change raise deeper questions. At some point, nations that devote ever more of their scarce resources of time, energy and capital to servicing the oldest members of their population, and extending their lives regardless of condition, must find this activity cutting into the resources available for both current consumption and future investment (Evans 1994).[15]

In any case, the health care services compete, within the public budget, with other programmes and institutions that can serve in different ways to mitigate the consequences of hierarchy and stress. Public budgets are under pressure everywhere, and health care systems, described by one observer as 'the hyaena gnawing on your foot', tend to have privileged access to such resources as are available. Whatever insights we may gain, from animal studies or elsewhere, about the determinants of health, the prospects of doing much about them are limited if this requires (public) money. Hypertrophy of the health care system thus has, in principle, the potential to be a hazard to health.[16]

On the other hand containment of health care costs tends in practice to be focused on the *public* services; expansion of the private sector has in recent years been treated with benign neglect. Yet the social gradient in health is real. Whether or not its sources lie beyond the reach of the health services, those services respond to real problems. Redirecting our health care systems so as to provide more services to those with lesser needs but greater incomes – which is what private systems inevitably do – seems questionable policy, to say the least.

Life is long, and the past is perpetually present

What then can be concluded from these studies? Well, a powerful advantage of studies of non-human primates is their ability to take a comprehensive view, both of the life cycle of the individual and of the social structure in which that life cycle is played out. Seen in that perspective, three features of health and hierarchy stand out that are relevant to human social policy:

- the existence of developmental 'windows of vulnerability';
- the length of the time periods over which the psychosocial environment has its effects; and
- the potential for the environment to buffer or compensate for both genetic vulnerabilities and physicochemical insults.

The observation of biological embeddedness clearly reinforces arguments for the importance of the experiences of very early life, and their potential influence over the whole of the life cycle. What happens in the year after (and the year before) birth can have permanent effects. This observation recalls the work of Barker et al. (1986; 1987; 1989; 1990), showing correlations between the health and circumstances of human infants at birth and during the first year, and mortality differences 50 years later.

But there are other windows. For the male animals, changing troops is a highly stressful time, exposing the psychological and physiological vulnerabilities of each individual. In some species adolescent males are routinely forced out of the natal troop, and some do not survive the re-entry process elsewhere. The parallel is obvious with the human transition to adulthood, and entry into the workforce, as a time of particular stress and risk with significant long-term consequences. Job change, likewise, has parallels with changing troops in mid-life, especially if one is forced out of one troop and must fight one's way into another. (Survival in isolation is, for social primates, a very dubious proposition.) Loss of employment, for adult male humans, is associated with increased risk of mortality (e.g. Morris et al. 1994).

Finally, the deterioration with age of the physiological mechanisms for coping with stress is found in a number of animal species. In later age a vicious circle is thus set up in which stress makes one more vulnerable to further stress. But the accumulated experiences of early life, both behavioural and biological, seem to exert a significant influence on the degree of vulnerability even in late age. The extension of these findings to humans is not yet clear, but it has recently become accepted that the level of education in early life is to some degree protective against Alzheimer's disease, decades later (Hertzman 1994).

Demonstrating long-term effects 'in the human' is difficult for both institutional and biological reasons. It is hard to keep research projects going for decades, and some of the subjects will outlive the investigators. But there are several long-term cohort studies whose study populations are moving into the age ranges at which significant health differentials might begin to appear. These may be of exceptional importance. And there is at least one striking example of a randomized trial of intervention in early life – the Perry High/ Scope Preschool Study – that has found very significant benefits 20 years later, effects that were not obvious in the early going (Schweinhart et al. 1993).[17]

Other shorter-term studies have shown that very early intervention programmes can compensate for a deprived rearing environment (e.g. Martin et al. 1990; Grantham-McGregor et al. 1991). There may, however, be a warning in some of the non-primate rearing studies reviewed by Cox. Infant monkeys separated from their mothers and reared by humans – a compensatory programme – do not show the depressed immune responses of those reared in isolation. But they do show other 'behavioural and central nervous system abnormalities' and 'increased susceptibility to gastrointestinal pathogens'.

It is thus possible that there is no true substitute for the real thing, and that social policy should be aimed at protecting and supporting the 'normal' primate-rearing environment, with compensatory programme, a second-best option. But this possibility could raise a great many difficult and politically explosive questions across the whole range of modern social and economic organization.

People are not, however, monkeys: over-enthusiastic extension of these findings to humans could be as misleading as failure to take them into account. For the moment, what can be said is that there is increasingly solid evidence, from both human and non-human primates, of biological effects on the individual from the psychosocial environment. These effects are potentially significant for the health of individuals; moreover, they appear to provide a biological foundation for observed differences in health status across the SES gradient in the population as a whole. Since these health gradients are large, in some societies at least, it follows that any measures that could equalize the health of the whole population to that of its most fortunate or successful members would have large health payoffs.

We do not at present know how to do this, and there is a real risk that effective policies, when we find them, will turn out to be too contentious and ideologically threatening to be acceptable. Indeed if they require a significant degree of sacrifice by some members of society, resistance will be quite understandable. But it must be recognized that continuous expansion of the care services also requires significant sacrifices (although the pattern of gainers and losers is different) in order to deal with the diseases and injuries that increasingly appear as the consequences, as much as the causes, of ill-health. The message from the animals is that a broader, more 'upstream' view of the determinants of health is biologically respectable as well as potentially more productive. At the very least we might be wise to spread our bets.

Notes

1. Left and Right are used here as labels for particular stylized perspectives, rather than groups of people. There are no doubt many who would identify themselves as Left, or Leftish, who are quite aware that material deprivation is not an adequate explanation of health experience in the developed societies. There are also doubtless Right-leaning people who go beyond the observation that some people are just 'better' than others, in all sorts of ways, to ask 'Why?' People on these paths risk convergence.

2. A recently published Canadian study, also person-specific and population-based, dwarfs even the Whitehall studies. Wolfson et al. (1993) examined the mortality experience of nearly half a million beneficiaries of the Canada Pension Plan, over the ten years following their retirement, and related this to their pre-retirement incomes as derived from tax records. Again a clear gradient emerges, with significantly higher probability of survival for those with higher incomes. Disability status is also recorded in the pension records; the result holds for those without reported disability.

3. The upward shift in the curve is interpreted by the authors of the *WDR* as reflecting improvements in other determinants of health, such as medical technology, public health, and public education and understanding of how to use available technologies.

4. This is misleading. In reality the principal problem is to obtain valid *basal* measures for each animal, which requires measures to be taken at the same time of day and season, avoiding animals that are sick or injured, or have just mated or been in a fight, or (for some purposes) eaten. Still, it would probably be difficult to dart one's civil servant just before breakfast or lunch, take him aside for a set of studies, and hold him in a cage overnight for recovery and release. Someone would notice, and eventually questions would be asked.

5. The 'fight or flight' response begins with, among other things, a rapid build-up of the adrenal hormone cortisol in the blood. A critical part of the control process is a feedback loop whereby the hypothalamus detects the level of circulating cortisol and regulates its rate of release. In subordinate animals the feedback 'signal' is weakened, so that the hypothalamus underestimates the level of circulating cortisol and production is not turned off appropriately. The subordinate animals consequently have higher basal levels of this hormone. In response to stress, however, the dominant animals can rapidly increase cortisol concentrations to levels equivalent to those in subordinates.

6. For the engineers, stresses are the external forces acting on a material or structure, and strain is the extent to which that material or structure is deformed, 'bent out of shape' as a result. 'Stressor' seems to have been introduced in those disciplines that have also used 'stress' to refer to the organism's physiological reactions to stress.

7. It is not possible among the baboons, as it is among the civil servants, to follow animals of different status through time and to compare standardized mortality rates and causes of death, because '...among [male baboons] ranks change over time and in idiosyncratic

ways'. This has not historically been true in the UK civil service; one does not lose status as physical powers fail. One might study the female baboons, whose status tends to be stable over the lifetime. But because mature female baboons spend much of their lives either pregnant or nursing, it would not be possible to anaesthetize them without risk to mother or baby.

8. Such measurements are not, of course, available to the student of free-living populations. Ethical and legal constraints discourage the removal of subjects' arteries for detailed analysis.

9. Interestingly Offord et al. (1989) found, in the Ontario child health study, that about 20 per cent of the child population suffered from some form of mental disorder.

10. Responses to stress are both physiological and behavioural. One probably should not draw too sharp a line between stress responses that are biologically embedded – in the endocrine system, e.g. – and those that are overtly behavioural – lighting up a cigarette, or getting drunk. How should one classify panic?

11. It is not clear to what extent anyone studying health inequalities actually holds the views that Charlton describes as 'The model implicit in work on health inequalities...' – his source is a publication from 1936. He assumes that health status *is* a mechanical function of (absolute) income, and claims that others do likewise. He then points out, correctly, that if the first differential of such a function is positive over its whole domain, rather than going to zero as income increases, then any redistribution of income must lower the health of losers while raising that of gainers. But Charlton seems to confuse the persistence of a positive first differential – no health plateau – with the existence of a non-negative second differential – no diminishing returns to income. The first does not imply the second. If the second differential is negative throughout the domain of the function, then total health will still be increased, on balance, by income redistribution. Charlton cites no evidence that the second differential is non-negative. The real problem, however, is that in affluent societies, the functional relationship between health and income is itself highly implausible.

12. This process shows up clearly in the present international movement for health care reform. In a time of declining economic expectations, some are concerned to improve the efficiency and effectiveness of health care systems. But others advocate various forms of 'privatization' simply to redistribute both access to care, and the burden of paying for it: more and better care for the (relatively) healthy and wealthy, at lower cost (in taxes), and less and poorer care, at greater cost (in charges), for the rest. Sharing is a luxury; 'we' cannot afford it now.

13. An exception to this broad generalization may be infant mortality rates, which do appear to have become much less unequal in some countries, but here the range of interventions goes beyond medical care narrowly defined.

14. Public health, however, is another matter (Szreter 1988).

15. There is increasing evidence to support what should in any case be obvious, that in many cases elderly people themselves do *not* want life-extending interventions in terminal care. But the decision has usually passed beyond their control.

16. We should obviously look first for signs of this in the US, where health care now takes up over 14 per cent of national income and is rising uncontrollably. But private versus public funding is almost certainly a red herring in this discussion. In the first place all modern health care systems depend, and must depend, primarily on public funding. Even in the US, while most people rely primarily upon private coverage, about half the costs come directly or indirectly from public funds. Second, even where significant amounts of funds flow through 'private' insurance channels, they are to the individual payroll deductions, job-related and largely involuntary, and look very much like taxes.

17. The Perry High/Scope Study actually demonstrates large improvements in the experimental group in social adjustment – school completion, job-holding and income, reduced rates of teenage pregnancy (females) and crime (males) – rather than health *per se*. But it is powerful evidence for the significance of long-term effects. One probably should not expect to observe health differences among a population still in their mid-twenties.

References

Baird, P.A. (1994), 'The Role of Genetics in Population Health' in Evans et al. (1994).

Barker, D.J.P., Bull, A.R., Osmond, C. and Simmonds, S.J. (1990), 'Fetal and placental size and risk of hypertension in adult life', *British Medical Journal*, **301**, 259–62.

Barker, D.J.P. and Osmond, C. (1987), 'Inequalities in health in Britain: Specific explanations in three Lancashire towns', *British Medical Journal*, **294**, 749–52.

Barker, D.J.P. and Osmond, C. (1986), 'Infant mortality, childhood nutrition and ischaemic heart disease in England and Wales', *The Lancet*, **i**, 1077–81.

Barker, D.J.P., Winter, P.D., Osmond, C., Margetts, B. and Simmonds, S.J. (1989), 'Weight in infancy and death from ischaemic heart disease', *The Lancet*, **ii**, 577–80.

Beardsley, T. (1994), 'A War Not Won', *Scientific American*, January, **270**(1), 130–38.

Bellinger, D., Leviton, A., Waternaux, C., Needleman, H. and Rabinowitz, M. (1993), 'Low-Level Lead Exposure, Social Class, and Infant Development', *Neurotoxicology and Teratology*, **10**, 497–503.

Charlton, B.G. (1994), 'Is inequality bad for the national health?', *The Lancet*, 22 January, **343**(8891), 221–2.

Cohen, S., Kaplan, J.R., Cunnick, J.E., Manuck, S.B. and Rabin, B.S. (1992), 'Chronic Social Stress, Affiliation, and Cellular Immune Response in Nonhuman Primates', *Psychological Science*, **3**(5), 301–4.

Cox, C.L. (1993), 'Psychosocial Factors and Immunity in Nonhuman Primates: A Review', *Psychosomatic Medicine*, **55**(3), 298–308.

Economist, The (1994a), 'The unhealthy poor', 4 June, pp. 55–6.

Economist, The (1994b), 'Peering into 2010: The Future of Medicine Survey', 19 March, pp. 3–18.

Evans, R.G., Barer, M.L. and Marmor, T.R. (eds) (1994), *Why Are Some People Healthy and Others Not? The Determinants of Health of Populations*, New York: Aldine–de Gruyter.

Evans, R.G. (1994), 'Health Care As a Threat to Health: Defence, Opulence, and the Social Environment', *Daedalus: Journal of the American Academy of Arts and Sciences*, Fall.

Grantham-McGregor, S.M., Powell, C.A., Walker, S.P. and Himes, J.H. (1991), 'Nutritional supplementation, psychosocial stimulation, and mental development of stunted children: the Jamaican study', *The Lancet*, 6 July, **338**(8758), 1–5.

Hamm, T.E. Jr, Kaplan, J.R., Clarkson, T.B. and Bullock, B.C. (1983), 'Effects of Gender and Social Behavior on the Development of Coronary Artery Atherosclerosis in Cynomolgous Macacques', *Atherosclerosis*, **48**, 221–33.

Hertzman, C. (1994), 'The Lifelong Impact of Childhood Experiences: a Population Health Perspective', *Daedalus: Journal of the American Academy of Arts and Sciences*, Fall.

Hertzman, C., Frank, J. and Evans, R.G. (1994), 'Heterogeneities in Health Status and the Determinants of Population Health' in Evans et al. (1994).

Kunst, A.E. and Mackenbach, J.P. (1992), *An international comparison of socio-economic inequalities in mortality*, Rotterdam: Department of Public Health and Social Medicine, Erasmus University, Rotterdam.

Marmot, M.G., Rose, G., Shipley, M. and Hamilton, P.J.S. (1978), 'Employment grade and coronary heart disease in British civil servants', *Journal of Epidemiology and Community Health*, **32**, 244–9.

Marmot, M.G. and Theorell, T. (1988), 'Class and cardiovascular disease: the contribution of work', *International Journal of Health Services*, **18**, 659–74.

Marmot, M.G. (1986), 'Social inequalities in mortality: the social environment' in Wilkinson, R.G. (ed.), *Class and Health*, London: Tavistock Publications, pp. 21–33.

Marmot, M.G., Davey Smith, G., Stansfeld, S., Patel, C., North, F., Head, J., White, I., Brunner, E. and Feeney A. (1991), 'Health Inequalities among British Civil Servants: the Whitehall II Study', *The Lancet*, 8 June, **337**, 1387–93.

Martin S.L., Ramey, C.T. and Ramey, S. (1990), 'The Prevention of Intellectual Impairment in Children of Impoverished Families: Findings of a Randomized Trial of Educational Day Care', *American Journal of Public Health*, **80**(7), 844–7.

McKeown T. (1979), *The role of medicine: dream, mirage, or nemesis?* Princeton: Princeton University Press.

Morris, J.K., Cook, D.G. and Shaper, A.G. (1994), 'Loss of Employment and Mortality', *British Medical Journal*, 30 April, **308**(6937), 1135–9.

North, F., Syme, S.L. Feeney, A. et al. (1993), 'Explaining socioeconomic differences in sickness absence: the Whitehall II Study', *British Medical Journal*, 6 February, **306**, 363.

Office of Population Censuses and Surveys (1978), *Occupational mortality: The Registrar General's decennial supplement for England and Wales, 1972*, Series DS No. 1, London: HMSO.

Offord, D.R., Boyle, M.H., Fleming, J.E., Blun, H.M. and Rae Grant, N.I. (1989), 'Ontario Child Health Study: Summary of Selected Results', *Canadian Journal of Psychiatry*, August, **34**(6), 483–91.

Preston, S.H. (1976), *Mortality Patterns in National Populations*, New York: Academic Press.

Sapolsky, R.M. (1990), 'Stress in the wild', *Scientific American*, **262**(1), 116–23.

Sapolsky, R.M. (1992), *Stress, the Aging Brain, and the Mechanisms of Neuron Death*, Cambridge, Mass.: The MIT Press.

Sapolsky R.M. (1993), 'Endocrinology Alfresco: Psychoendocrine Studies of Wild Baboons', *Recent Progress in Hormone Research*, **48**, 437–68.

Schweinhart, L.J., Barnes, H.V. and Weikart, D.P. (1993), *Significant Benefits: The High/Scope Perry Preschool Study Through Age 27*, Ypsilanti, Michigan: The High/Scope Press.

Stoddart, G.L. and Lavis J. (1994), 'Can We Have Too Much Health Care?', *Daedalus: Journal of the American Academy of Arts and Sciences*, Fall.

Suomi, S.J. (1991), 'Primate Separation Models of Affective Disorders' in Madden, J. (ed.), *Neurobiology of Learning, Emotion and Affect*, New York: Raven Press.

Szreter, S. (1988), 'The Importance of Social Intervention in Britain's Mortality Decline *c.* 1850–1914: a Re-interpretation of the Role of Public Health', *The Society for the Social History of Medicine*, **1**(1), 1–37.

Townsend, P. and Davidson, N. (eds) (1988), 'The Black Report' in *Inequalities in Health*, London: Penguin, pp. 29–213.

Vågerö D. and Lundberg, O. (1989), 'Health inequalities in Britain and Sweden', *The Lancet*, 1 July, **ii**, 35–6.

Werner, E.E. (1989a), 'Children of the Garden Isle', *Scientific American*, **260**(4) (April), 106–11.

Werner, E.E. (1989b), 'High Risk Children in Young Adulthood: A Longitudinal Study from Birth to 32 Years', *American Journal of Orthopsychiatry*, January, **59**(1), 72–81.

Werner E.E. and Smith, R.S. (1982), *Vulnerable but invincible: a longitudinal study of resilient children and youth*, New York: McGraw-Hill.

Wilkins R. and Adams, O. (1983), *The Healthfulness of Life*, Montreal: The Institute for Research on Public Policy.

Wilkinson, R.G. (1986), 'Socio-economic differences in mortality: interpreting the data on their size and trends' in Wilkinson, R.G. (ed.), *Class and Health*, London: Tavistock Publications, pp. 1–20.

Wilkinson, R.G. (1992), 'Income Distribution and Life Expectancy', *British Medical Journal*, **304**, 165–8.

Wolfson M., Rose, G., Gentleman, J.F. and Tomiak, M. (1993), 'Career Earnings and Death: A Longitudinal Analysis of Older Canadian Men', *Journal of Gerontology: Social Sciences*, July, **48**(4), S167–S179.

World Bank (1993), *World Development Report 1993: Investing in Health*, New York: Oxford University Press for the World Bank.

4 Contracts and competition in the NHS*

Martin Chalkley and James M. Malcomson

Introduction

One key element in the recent reforms of the NHS is the separation of *purchasers* from *providers*. The health authorities that receive funds from the government to arrange for health services to be provided are now separate organizations from the hospitals, clinics, etc. who actually care for patients. The provision of services is governed by *contracts* between those purchasers and providers. A second key element is that there should be *competition* between providers so that no hospital can be sure that it will always get the contract to provide, for example, hip and joint replacements in a particular area of the country unless it provides a competitive service. These two key elements are seen as linked – competition is more genuine if none of the competing providers is part of the same organization as the purchaser.

The purpose of these reforms is to provide a better health service. Whether or not they will do that is a broad question, to which we would expect an answer only as the result of experience. It nevertheless makes sense to ask the more limited questions of *what effects increased competition might have* and, if there is to be separation between purchasers and providers, *how the kinds of contracts used influence the health services delivered.* These are the questions with which this chapter is concerned.

We first consider the potential roles for competition between providers, how significant these are likely to be for the NHS, and the implications of the recent reforms for these roles. Our general conclusion is that the role traditionally seen for competition in limiting the economic inefficiency associated with monopoly power is unlikely to be fundamental to the NHS, at least in its present form. Of more importance, as those employed in health authorities become more and more distanced from their former responsibility for the direct provision of services, is likely to be the role of competitive tendering in providing information both about the prices at which services can actually be delivered and about which providers can deliver those services at the lowest prices.

*The support of the Economic and Social Research Council (ESCR) is gratefully acknowledged. The work was part of the ESRC Contracts and Competition Research Programme and was funded by ESRC award number L114251005. We are grateful to Tony Culyer, Ray Robinson and participants in both the British Association meeting and the ESRC Contracts and Competition programme workshop held at Robinson College, Cambridge, 19–20 September 1994, for helpful comments and discussions.

There is of course much more to ensuring adequate health care provision than simply achieving the lowest overall cost to a health authority. With services like health care for which it is not easy to monitor all aspects of the *quality* of the service provided, there is a real danger that awarding a contract to the lowest bidder will result in degradation of quality. It is here that contracts between providers and purchasers have a vital role to play. Contracts have to be designed carefully to maintain quality of service at acceptable levels. We discuss ways to do this in a later section. We argue there that the most appropriate form of contract depends on the extent to which quality can be assessed by patients and on how much the particular provider actually cares about the quality of services delivered to patients. We relate our conclusions to the kinds of contracts that have been used in practice.

When some potential providers care less than others, encouraging bidding for contracts raises a problem that we discuss in a further section. If contracts are awarded to the lowest bidder, there is a risk that the quality of services will be driven down to below the level that the health authority would wish to see provided. This raises a question regarding the possible alternative ways of ensuring quality.

One alternative to maintaining quality standards by contract is to rely on the reputations of providers. If those who provide good quality services are rewarded by having their contracts renewed whereas those suspected of skimping on quality do not, there can be a strong incentive to provide high quality. This will only work, however, if contracts have a relatively short duration – without that, the threat not to renew becomes less powerful. We therefore consider how the use of short-term contracts gives rise to its own problems, in particular what are known as the *ratchet* and *hold-up* effects that result in higher costs and less investment in new methods and equipment.

Before we discuss these ideas in detail, a few remarks about the framework we use are in order. We do not discuss how the budgets of health authorities are, or should be, determined. That is an issue discussed elsewhere in this book. We simply start from the undoubted fact that these budgets are not (and are never likely to be) enough for health authorities to purchase all the health services they would like to purchase. Nor do we discuss how health authorities should, or do, decide on what services are to have priority given their limited budgets – again that is an issue discussed elsewhere. The issues of concern here are the implications of competition for the cost and quality of the services provided and how contracts and competition can be used to meet the priorities that have been set with a limited budget.

One criterion we discuss is *economic efficiency*. It is important to understand the precise sense in which this term is used. Economic efficiency is concerned with the health authority getting as far down the list of priorities as possible for a given level of reward to the providing organization and the people who work for it. (*Reward* here is to be interpreted broadly to include non-monetary, as well as monetary, rewards.) It would not be economically efficient if, for example, a health authority were prepared to pay more for some service than the *minimum* a hospital would accept to provide it but the service was not in fact purchased. Economic efficiency is *not* synonymous with reducing costs, driving wages down, or many of the other senses in which the term efficiency has been used in debates on the NHS.

In this respect economic efficiency is different from *budgetary efficiency*, which is concerned solely with getting as far down the list of priorities as possible given a limited budget. Budgetary efficiency necessarily entails economic efficiency because an improvement in economic efficiency always enables the health authority to get further down its list of priorities for a given budget. But budgetary efficiency also entails driving down costs wherever possible by reducing the rewards to those providing services, something a health authority may be keen to do. We emphasize the difference between these concepts of efficiency because arguments based purely on economic efficiency are likely to be less controversial than those that make use of the additional criteria in budgetary efficiency.[1]

Our final introductory remark concerns terminology. For concreteness, we often refer to purchasers of health care as health authorities and to providers as hospitals. What we say about the latter, however, applies equally well to other types of providers, such as community health trusts, nursing homes, and so on.

Competition

There are different interpretations of the word competition. In everyday language, competition is often taken to mean sellers pursuing active strategies against each other – advertising, price cutting, sales promotions and the marketing of new and better products are seen as reflecting fierce competition. Here we use the word in its standard economic sense to refer to the number and type of actual and potential suppliers of a service. The limiting case is *perfect competition* where each supplier is individually powerless to influence the price at which services are provided because of the large number of other potential suppliers.

In general, we see four potential roles for competition: reducing the economic inefficiencies that arise from monopoly power; reducing the influence providers have over purchasers' decisions; ensuring customers receive the types of products and services they want; and providing information to purchasers about the prices at which suppliers *can* provide products and services so that they get what they want at the lowest cost. In this section, we discuss in turn the extent to which each of these applies to the recent reforms of the NHS.

Competition, monopoly power and economic inefficiency

There is a large literature that investigates the relationship between the *competitiveness* of supply (the number and types of suppliers) and *performance* (measured by quantity sold) compared to what would happen if supply were perfectly competitive. This literature is reviewed extensively in Tirole (1989). Perfect competition is used as a benchmark for these comparisons because, under certain conditions, it results in an economically efficient level of sales. Typically, economic models predict that greater competition (a greater number of competing suppliers) leads to performance closer to the perfectly competitive benchmark. At the other extreme a single (monopoly) supplier chooses a higher price than under perfect competition and, as a result, sales are inefficiently low. It is this prediction that is widely regarded as providing a case for increased competition and that forms the basis of much government competition policy.

The underlying argument is as follows. Perfect competition results in a price that reflects the *marginal cost* of an extra sale (the additional cost to the supplier of supplying one extra sale). This happens because it is in the interest of each individual supplier to continue to expand sales until the price received just covers the cost of supplying the last unit. In deciding how much to buy, customers consider whether an extra unit is worth the price. But when price is equal to marginal cost, they are in effect considering whether an extra unit is worth the cost of supplying it. A health purchaser who, for example, decides on three extra hip replacements rather than an extra coronary bypass operation on the basis of what a hospital charges is then actually choosing on the basis of what it really entails in terms of resources to carry out the operations. Moreover, if the price of everything is equal to its marginal cost, it cannot be that a customer would prefer to have something else *unless it costs more to supply*. But if it costs more to supply, some other customer would, since resources are limited, necessarily be disadvantaged by the switch. One customer's interest can be advanced only by harming some other.

Critical to this argument is that individual suppliers cannot influence the price at which they can sell. If, however, there is a single supplier, that will not be the case. A single supplier can choose whether to sell a little at a high price or more at a lower price. The most profitable choice will be when an additional sale generates as much revenue (*marginal revenue*) as it adds to cost. But marginal revenue is lower than price because, to sell more, the supplier has to lower the price. The additional revenue from cutting the price to achieve an extra sale is thus the price at which that sale is made *less* the amount by which the revenue from all other sales is reduced because the price is lower. Since the most profitable choice of sales is where marginal revenue equals marginal cost and price is greater than marginal revenue, it follows that price is above marginal cost. Thus, when customers base their decisions on prices, these decisions do not necessarily reflect the actual costs of supply – a customer might prefer something different that actually costs no more to supply because prices are not equal to marginal costs. It will then in general be possible to advance one customer's interests without harming those of any others (and, indeed, even the interest of the monopolist) – a classic case of economic inefficiency.

The essence of this analysis is that, in order to capture the profits made possible by monopoly power, a monopoly supplier sets price above marginal cost. Since customers base their decisions on prices, those decisions are not then based on the actual costs of supply. In many cases, including health services, the actual cost of supply is not known in advance, so a price set in advance cannot be set precisely equal to marginal cost. What perfect competition ensures in this case is that price is set at the lowest level at which the supplier is willing to undertake to supply in view of the uncertainty in costs. This price is termed the supplier's *reservation price*. But the substance of the argument continues to apply if we replace the term *marginal cost* by the term *reservation price*.

This argument for the economic inefficiency of monopoly hinges on customers simply accepting that the price quoted by the supplier is the price that has to be paid and basing their purchasing decisions on that. This is typically true for individual shoppers in a supermarket. It is certainly not true for health authorities which can, and do, bargain over what they will pay for services. It is well known, for example, that the central buying power of the NHS has enabled it to bargain for prices for drugs supplied to the NHS that are lower than in many other countries.

Where purchasers are active in negotiating prices, there are more efficient arrangements they can reach with a monopoly supplier than simply paying the monopoly price. A purchaser could, for example, offer to pay the reservation price plus a lump sum that ensures the supplier's profits are no less than at the monopoly price. (Some of the cost and volume contracts negotiated between health authorities and NHS hospitals involve what amounts to a lump sum in addition to a price for each treatment.) The supplier would then make as much profit as at the monopoly price and the purchaser would have the advantage of the additional treatments that it regards as cost-effective at the supplier's reservation price but not at the monopoly price. The economic efficiency properties of perfect competition would then apply because price would be equal to the reservation price, despite there being only a single supplier. Budgetary efficiency would, in addition, involve reducing the lump sum as far as possible while still getting the service supplied.

Such mutually advantageous economically efficient arrangements are always *possible* when purchasers and providers negotiate over the terms of supply but that does not necessarily mean they will actually come about. The supplier would still make more profit supplying for a slightly lower lump sum than not supplying at all. The health authority, in pursuit of budgetary efficiency, would like to reduce the total outlay so that it can use the savings to purchase other health services and will therefore try to bargain down the amount of the lump sum. The supplier will bargain to resist this. Will the outcome of their bargaining be economically efficient and how much will the purchaser actually end up paying?

A standard way of answering these questions is with game-theoretic models of bargaining. Gibbons (1992) and Binmore (1992) provide accessible discussions of these. A typical conclusion from this literature is that, provided the purchaser and the supplier know enough about each other, they will settle for an outcome that is as good as possible for the purchaser without harming the interest of the supplier. (There are some bargaining arrangements that may result in other outcomes but for obvious reasons both purchaser and supplier have every interest in avoiding these.) The essential reasoning is as follows. Suppose the purchaser knows the lowest price (the reservation price) at which the provider is prepared to sell any given number and quality of treatments and the provider knows what the purchaser is prepared to pay for any given number and quality of treatments. If the purchaser were prepared to pay more for an additional treatment than the supplier's reservation price, the purchaser would gain without the supplier losing by having that treatment supplied at a price equal to the reservation price. If the supplier must be given part of the gain to be persuaded to agree, that can be achieved by an increase in the lump sum so that they *both* gain. Thus both their interests will be served by always settling for an outcome with the number and quality of treatments that the purchaser is prepared to pay for at the reservation price and bargaining over the lump sum to decide how the gains will be divided. But a change in the lump sum to the advantage of one party can only be at the expense of the other. Thus the bargained outcome will always have the property that the purchaser's position cannot be improved without the supplier being disadvantaged, precisely the criterion for economic efficiency in the provision of the service.

The conclusion we draw from this discussion is that, even with monopoly supply, it is not necessary to introduce competition to prevent the *economic* inefficiency associated with monopoly power, provided (as in the NHS as currently constituted) the purchaser and supplier bargain over the prices of the services to be provided. That might change if, for example, a single hospital group were to buy up a chain of hospitals that formed a significant part of the UK market. It might also change as purchasers become more fragmented through the continued growth of GP fundholding. There are, however, other mechanisms for dealing with such issues. Indeed, a mechanism to counteract the fragmented purchasing power of GP fundholders is already developing in the form of purchasing consortia that negotiate with providers on behalf of groups of GP practices. Competition might, of course, still improve *budgetary* efficiency if it increases the bargaining power of purchasers relative to providers. That, however, is a different issue from the economic inefficiency traditionally associated with monopoly. We take up that issue in a later section.

Crucial to the argument just presented is that the health authority and the hospital know sufficient about, respectively, the price at which the hospital is prepared to provide treatments and the amount the health authority is prepared to pay. Without that, bargaining between them may not result in an efficient settlement. To see why, suppose the health authority does not know the price at which the provider is prepared to supply. By pretending that it requires a higher price than it actually does, the hospital may induce the health authority to pay more than it needs to. So the hospital may have an interest in hiding the price at which it is prepared to supply treatments. Similarly, the health authority may have an interest in hiding how much it is really willing to pay. Unless bargaining reveals the truth, they may not settle on an outcome with the number and quality of treatments that the health authority would be prepared to pay for if priced at the reservation price simply because neither of them knows what that number and quality are. The outcome will not then be economically efficient.

This economic inefficiency is somewhat different from the inefficiency traditionally associated with monopoly power. In essence, it arises from lack of information. Lack of information about the reservation prices of suppliers may also prevent the health authority from achieving provision of services at the lowest cost (budgetary efficiency). We discuss the role competition may play in providing information later. But before we do that we discuss two further roles for competition: first, in reducing the ability of providers to influence purchasers' decisions; and second, in helping to ensure that patients receive the services they really want.

Competition and provider influence over purchasers
The above analysis presumes that health authorities decide their priorities for services independently of the providers. But those individuals responsible for making purchasing decisions may be subject to pressures that affect their decisions. There are interest groups, including the providing institutions themselves, who may like to influence health care purchasing decisions in their private interests. Such groups may attempt to influence purchasers. If they are successful, the public interest may be perverted. Even if unsuccessful, they may use up valuable resources in the process of trying to obtain influence. This is an issue whenever the conduct of public policy, whether the purchasing of health care or the regulation of monopolized industries, is entrusted to

individuals who may be susceptible to influence by interest groups. It has been analysed extensively in the case of regulatory bodies, in which it is known as *regulatory capture*. Laffont and Tirole (1993, Chap. 11) discuss this issue in detail.

One argument that has been made for increasing competition between suppliers to the NHS is that it breaks down the close personal relationships between employees of the purchaser and those of the provider, thus reducing the influence that providers have over the decisions of purchasers. We know of no formal argument that demonstrates this. However, even if it is correct, there is another aspect to this issue. Suppliers who compete to influence a purchaser in their favour use up resources in doing so. There is a substantial literature on such *rent-seeking* behaviour. See Nitzan (1994) for a survey. That literature suggests that competition between rent-seekers is an extremely wasteful process. The resulting waste must be set against any gains from distancing providers from purchasers.

Competition and patient satisfaction

There is a common perception that where there is a lack of competition, customers have to accept the kinds of products and services that suppliers choose to offer. In contrast, competition between suppliers ensures that suppliers offer the kinds of products and services that customers really want. An obvious comparison is between the reputation for limited range, poor quality and shoddy service under Soviet central planning and the sometimes bewildering variety on offer in some Western economies. At root, this would seem closely related to the use of monopoly power as discussed above. After all, as Hicks put it, the best of all monopoly profits is an easy life. However, the argument presented above implicitly took as given the nature of what was being supplied. It was not concerned with the effect of competition on the range on offer and on how that might change over time as one supplier tries to steal a competitive march on the others by designing a new and better product.

There has been a certain amount of discussion of these issues in the literature. See, for example, Lancaster (1979). It is not at all clear, however, that this is relevant in the context of the NHS. A characteristic of the NHS is that purchasers decide what services are to be made available to patients – it is not patients themselves who decide this. Under the recent reforms, purchasing authorities have been told to actively seek the views of local people before deciding their priorities for health care spending. But there is no inherent connection between consulting with users and the separation of purchasers from providers. Nor is it obvious why competition between suppliers should have the effect of meeting patients' needs more closely when the decisions on purchasing are made by a health authority and the continued prosperity of the suppliers depends primarily on satisfying that health authority.

Health authorities are not, however, the only purchasers in the reformed NHS. Fundholding GPs also purchase services on behalf of patients. If GPs are more responsive to what their patients want than health authorities, or if patients are in a position to switch between GPs until they find one who is responsive to what they want, then the reforms may result in the supply of services being more closely aligned to what patients want. Any such effect would, of course, have more to do with competition between purchasers for patients than with competition between suppliers. Whether or not such an effect will come about seems to depend crucially on the terms under which patients can switch GPs and the response of GPs to patients who want to switch. These are issues on which others have more expertise than we do.

Competition and information

The argument we have presented above for bargaining resulting in an outcome that is economically efficient depends on the parties having sufficient information about each other. In particular, it relies on the purchaser knowing the reservation price at which the supplier is prepared to provide a service and the supplier knowing how much the purchaser is really prepared to pay for that service. Differences in what the purchaser and supplier know may well increase over time in the NHS as the hitherto close relationships between provider and purchaser become more remote. Competition can help to provide the parties with information but, before we discuss how, it is helpful to explain precisely why the lack of information may result in the bargained outcome being economically inefficient. An example demonstrates this.

Suppose a health authority, in view of its limited budget, decides that it is prepared to pay a hospital up to £B for a particular treatment and that the hospital decides it really cannot afford to carry out the treatment for less than £C (so £C is its reservation price), where $B > C$ so that there is certainly a price for the treatment at which both would like it to go ahead. Suppose also that the hospital knows both B and C but that the health authority knows only B. The health authority wants the treatment carried out but it would also like to keep the cost down so that the savings can be used for other treatments. The hospital would like to keep the price high so that it can, for example, afford some new equipment for treating other patients. If the hospital is in a position to dictate the price, it will specify a price of £B (which it knows) and the treatment will be carried out. If the health authority is in a position to dictate price, it has to consider two things. If it offers a price of £B, the treatment will certainly be carried out but it will have no savings to use elsewhere. If it offers a lower price, the treatment will be carried out if the price is above £C and it will have some savings to use elsewhere. But if the price turns out to be below £C, the hospital will refuse to carry out the treatment. That outcome is economically inefficient – both parties would prefer the treatment to be carried out at some price between £C and £B but the lack of information prevents them reaching agreement.

In the example given, it is always possible to ensure the treatment is carried out by letting the hospital set the price, the procedure implicit in the NHS Management Executive guidelines. (See Dawson 1994 and Ferguson and Palmer 1994 for discussions of those guidelines.) Although the health authority may not be happy at how much it has to pay, it is always *possible*, in this simple example, to achieve an efficient outcome. But even that may not be the case if the hospital does not know B. In particular, if it is not known for sure that $B > C$, there exists no bargaining procedure that ensures treatment will always be carried out promptly whenever $B > C$. (There may be a way of ensuring that, if they bargain long enough, the treatment will *eventually* be carried out whenever $B > C$, but this too is not economically efficient because it imposes additional suffering on patients awaiting treatment.) The classic statement of this result is Myerson and Satterthwaite (1983).

It is the lack of information that generates the inefficiency. But, if there are many hospitals capable of carrying out the treatment, competition between them can reveal information about the prices at which they would be prepared to carry out treatments. A common form of competition for public services is *competitive tendering* – any supplier who wishes can put in a bid for providing the service and the contract is awarded to the lowest bidder. Standard auction and bidding theory (for example, McAfee and McMillan 1987) tells us a great deal about the outcome of such competitive tendering. A standard result is that, if the suppliers have different reservation prices at which they are prepared to provide the service, the contract will go to the supplier with the lowest reservation price at a price that is, on average, just below the reservation price of the supplier with the second lowest reservation price. This is seen most easily in what is called an *English auction*, in which bidding continues, with the bids being known by all participants, until all but one of the bidders has dropped out of the bidding. The supplier with the second lowest reservation price will drop out once the price has been bid down below its reservation price. That will leave the supplier with the lowest reservation price committed to providing the service at a price just slightly below the reservation price of the second lowest bidder. With a *sealed bid competitive tender* (in which suppliers make bids that are unknown to the other bidders and the purchaser takes the lowest bid), the winning bid may turn out higher or lower than with an English auction but on average it is exactly the same.

Bidding for contracts thus reveals (at least on average) the price at which the second lowest bidder is prepared to provide the service. As long as the purchaser is prepared to pay at least that for the service, it will be provided. Bidding therefore reduces the extent of the economic inefficiency associated with bargaining discussed above. Moreover increased competition, in the form of more bidders, on average reduces the price that the purchaser has to pay (see McAfee and McMillan 1987, p. 711). In that way it also promotes budgetary efficiency. The essential intuition is that the more bidders there are, the lower on average is the price the second lowest bidder is prepared to accept. Thus increased competition has two advantages for the purchaser. First, it contributes to economic efficiency by reducing the likelihood of the service not being provided when the purchaser does not know the reservation price of a provider. Second, it contributes to budgetary efficiency by lowering the price that the purchaser has to pay.

But getting the service provided at the lowest price may not be such a good idea if the lowest-price service is also a lower-quality service. Ensuring that this does not happen is a serious issue in bidding for health services, as indeed for many other public services. The reason is that specifying and monitoring the quality of the service to be provided is not straightforward. If competitive bidding is to lead to a *good*, as well as a cheap, service the contracts offered for tender must be designed carefully to maintain quality. We discuss what can be done in the next section.

Contracts

Contract enforcement

Contracts between purchasers and providers are used to govern the quantity and quality of the health services provided. But what can be achieved by contract is limited by what can be enforced, by going to court if necessary. Contract provisions may be unenforceable because they are not regarded as legally binding. That is the case with contracts between two NHS bodies (though not between, say, a health authority and a privately run nursing home) because the National Health Service and Community Care Act (1990) specifically states that these contracts are not subject to contract law. (There are other branches of the law under which *NHS contracts*, as these are known, might still be enforceable. See Barker 1993, 1995 for a discussion of this issue.) For NHS contracts there is, however, an arbitration procedure that replaces enforcement by contract law.

What the parties intend to happen under a contract may also not be enforced because a court (or arbitrator) does not have the information to enforce it. It might seem that the parties could deal with this by ensuring that the contract is clear. But it is not that simple. Even contracts that are drawn up carefully may remain obscure. The parties may not have envisaged some possibilities, so no provision is made for them. Even if they do envisage all the possibilities, it may just be too costly or time-consuming to write all the relevant details into a contract. And even if they would like to write all the relevant details into a contract, they may be unable to do so in such a way that a court can enforce their intention. The first two of these are self-explanatory. An example may be useful to clarify the third. It may simply not be possible to describe sufficiently precisely in a contract the circumstances in which a health authority wants a particular medical procedure to be carried out in such a way that, if a dispute arises over whether that procedure should have been carried out, a court (or arbitrator) can verify months later whether those circumstances actually applied to a particular patient. Faced with a dispute, it is the job of the court or arbitrator to make a judgement one way or the other but the judgement may not be what the parties would have written into the contract had they been able to do so. When the information needed to enforce the parties' intentions is available to the court or arbitrator, that information is said to be *verifiable*.

In practice, lack of verifiability is a serious issue in contracting for health services. This is particularly true for those aspects of a contract that are concerned with the quality of service. Conventions on medical malpractice set certain minimum standards but these may well be substantially below the standards a health authority would like. Somewhat higher standards may be enforced by careful monitoring and documentation to ensure the relevant information is verifiable. But, since monitoring the quality of services is costly and time-consuming, a health authority cannot possibly hope to monitor the quality of service provided for each patient treated. The best it can hope to do in practice is check up on the services provided to a small number of patients by a quality assurance procedure. Where it is costly to make relevant information verifiable, it may make sense to design contracts that do not rely on verifiability. It is to the design of such contracts that we now turn. In discussing contract design, we use the term *quality* as a shorthand for those dimensions of a service that are of concern to purchasers and that the parties to the contract either cannot enforce by contract or for which they decide not to set up the costly mechanism to enable them to do so.

Contracting for quality of service

A major issue in contracting for health services is ensuring that an appropriate quality of service is provided while maintaining incentives for hospitals to keep costs under control. Central to this is how a hospital responds to a particular contract. That in turn depends partly on the extent to which patients both correctly perceive the quality of treatment that a hospital offers and are in a position to respond in choosing where they are treated.

If only one aspect of quality matters and patients respond quickly to that in their choice of where they seek treatment, the health authority can achieve precisely the level of quality it would like to achieve, while retaining economically efficient incentives to keep costs under control, by paying the hospital a fixed price per patient treated (a *cost per case contract*, or in US terminology a *prospective payment* system); see Ma (1994). The intuition for this is that hospitals get paid more by attracting more patients and do this by increasing the quality of service they provide until the cost of providing additional quality offsets the price per treatment. By appropriate choice of price, the health authority can induce any level of quality it wishes. Moreover, with a fixed price per case, the hospital retains any cost savings it makes and so has an incentive to keep costs down.

In practice, there are many important aspects to quality such as quality of medical services, quality of nursing services, quality of hotel services, and many more. In Chalkley and Malcomson (1995a), we show that the same conclusion applies in this case but only if patients perceive *every* aspect of the quality of service correctly and respond to all those aspects. Patient demand then keeps all aspects of quality in line even when patients do not themselves pay for the services they receive. This result emphasizes the importance of providing information about quality to patients, or at least to the GPs who guide their choices of where to be treated. But it also indicates the limitation of using this mechanism to ensure quality. As has been emphasized certainly since Arrow's seminal (1963) article, health care is a service for which there are particular problems in ensuring that patients know as much as providers about the outcomes of the services they receive.

There are also other problems with relying on this mechanism. First, for hospitals that have long waiting lists for treatment, little incentive to provide quality in order to attract yet more patients is provided by a payment that is received only when the cases are actually treated. Second, patients may not be in a position to choose where they are treated on the basis of their perceptions of quality. This is particularly true for patients whose treatment is paid for by a health authority that has a contract with only one provider for that treatment. Third, some aspects of quality (*experience*, as opposed to *search*, aspects of quality in the jargon) can be assessed only while being treated. For many health services, an individual patient does not receive frequent treatment, so that the patient's own demand is not affected by the quality received. The demand for services is then affected by quality only through the effects of reputation and only in the future, which may temper a hospital's incentive to provide those aspects of quality.

The first of these problems can be overcome by making part of the payment for each patient payable at the time a patient is added to the waiting list. By appropriate choice of payment, the health authority can then provide exactly the same incentives for the hospital to provide quality as when there is no waiting list. The second, however, seems fundamental to NHS services purchased by health authorities (in contrast to those purchased by GP fundholders). The third seems fundamental to any system of providing health services. It is thus important to consider ways in which contracts can ensure high-quality services when patient demand will not do so.

In discussing this issue, we should distinguish between hospitals with different objectives. One possible hospital objective discussed in the literature is maximizing profit. But we must remember that, even in the US, there are substantial numbers of hospitals that are non-profit institutions alongside hospitals that operate for profit. For understanding the contracting issues that arise when demand does not respond to quality, it is instructive to consider three different types of objectives hospitals may have. The first is pure *self-interest*. This is not synonymous with maximizing profit. Non-profit institutions can be equally self-interested (about, for example, the perks and the power of those who run them). But some hospitals are no doubt *benevolent* in the sense that they genuinely want to do what is best for their patients for its own sake, not just because of the contractual consequences. Given a budget to spend freely, such a hospital will spend it on its patients in exactly the way a health authority that has its patients' interests at heart would want the hospital to spend it. A hospital cannot, though, be expected to know the health authority's priorities for care purchased from other hospitals and so even a benevolent hospital may choose to spend all its budget on its *own* patients. (Since our brief here is not concerned with how the priorities of health authorities reflect those of patients, in what follows we discuss 'benevolence' solely with respect to the health authority's priorities.) These cases are extremes – but extremes are useful for isolating analytical issues. Between them lies what we term a *partially benevolent* hospital that gives some weight to the goals of the health authority but also gives some weight to its own self-interest. Even with the best will in the world, it is only natural that hospital employees have their own particular concerns.

At first sight, it might seem that there would be no contracting problems with benevolent hospitals even if the demand for their services does not respond to the quality they provide: given a budget to spend freely, they would choose to do what the health authority would want them to do, so why not just give them the money and let them get on with it? But there is the question of *how much* money to give them. If they are given a fixed amount to treat patients with a particular diagnosis (a *block contract*, as it has come to be known) but the number of patients to be treated turns out to be larger than expected, the hospital will not have enough money to treat them all. It may end up closing wards towards the end of the financial year (a familiar characteristic in UK hospitals in recent times) because it has run out of money to treat non-emergency patients as the result of treating a great many patients earlier in the year. If, on the other hand, the hospital is given enough money to treat the maximum number of patients to be treated under any circumstances and there turn out to be fewer than that, the health authority will have used up funds that it might have preferred to use elsewhere. With a benevolent hospital, a block contract will work well where the number of patients to be treated is known in advance – for example, non-emergency procedures for which capacity for treatment is limited and always fully utilized.

Where (as is obviously the case with emergency procedures) the number to be treated is not known in advance, ensuring that the hospital has just enough money to treat the appropriate number of patients can be achieved only if the amount it receives depends on the number to be treated, that is, the demand for its services. It might seem that an appropriate form of contract would then be to pay the hospital the cost of treating patients to the desired quality level for each patient treated. However, even with a benevolent hospital, that can distort the hospital's treatment decisions. The reason is subtle. Because a benevolent hospital has the same objectives for its patients as the health authority, it will make the decisions that the health authority would want it to make about how to spend a *fixed* budget on them. But, if it receives a payment for *each* patient treated, it can increase its budget by treating more patients. Since it would always like to have more funds (to, for example, treat more non-emergency patients so as to reduce its waiting lists), it has an incentive to treat too many patients with a somewhat cheaper service so that it can treat more patients in total. The detailed argument is given in Chalkley and Malcomson (1995b). One way to avoid this is to pay the hospital a fixed amount plus, for each patient treated, the cost of treatment at the desired quality level, but only up to the maximum number of patients the health authority would like to have treated given the length of the waiting list. This is one form of what is called a *cost and volume contract*. This discussion emphasizes the importance of putting a maximum on the number of patients to be treated in non-emergency categories (a maximum that may depend on the number wanting treatment) even with a benevolent hospital whose goals do not conflict with those of the health authority.

Now consider the other extreme, a self-interested hospital. If the demand for its services does not respond to the quality it provides, a purely self-interested hospital will always skimp on unverifiable quality unless its actual costs in providing high-quality services are directly reimbursed. There are two difficulties with achieving quality by cost reimbursement. First, it must be possible to verify what the actual costs of a particular treatment are. Second, even if actual costs can be verified, it is not straightforward to establish whether those costs were actually necessary to achieve the desired quality. With a purely self-interested hospital there is thus a dilemma. Either costs are reimbursed, in which case high-quality services may be provided but with the risk that costs will soar, as with the cost reimbursement rules previously used for Medicare in the US. Or costs are not reimbursed, in which case there is a strong incentive for the hospital to keep costs down but quality will suffer. The only way to overcome this dilemma is by auditing procedures that make quality verifiable – there is nothing, short of specifying in detail what is to be done under each set of circumstances and monitoring it, that the design of a contract can do to help.

If the health authority decides to go for cost-saving, the best that can be done is to pay the hospital a lump sum plus, for each case treated, a fixed amount that is independent of the number of cases treated. This takes us back to a *cost per case* contract or *prospective payment* system. The fixed amount per case treated should reflect the amount the health authority is prepared to pay for treating an additional patient at the quality level it can actually get the hospital to supply with the auditing procedures it has available. The economic intuition for this is as follows. Faced with a fixed payment per case, a self-interested hospital will always take full account of the costs of providing treatment. What the contract has to induce it to take account of is what the health authority regards as the benefit of treatment. Faced with the cost per case contract just described, it will treat patients up to the point at which the benefit from treating an additional patient (as reflected in the health authority's view about how much it is prepared to pay for the quality of service that will actually be delivered) just covers the additional cost. But unless quality can be enforced by effective auditing procedures, the quality of services will be lower than the health authority would choose if it could ensure that the chosen quality would be delivered.

We come now to the third type of hospital, a partially benevolent hospital. There are two forces pushing a hospital in the direction of benevolence. One is a natural concern for the welfare of patients, even if that concern is not so strong as to completely swamp self-interest. That is a genuine case of partial benevolence. The second is not what one would normally think of as benevolence but has very much the same implications for the present analysis. Even if quality cannot be enforced by audit procedures, the hospital may be concerned that, if it delivers low-quality services, word will get around, its reputation will suffer and, as a result, it will get fewer cases to treat in the future and possibly worse terms out of the health authority in any future contract negotiations. We discuss reputations in more detail in the next section. What is relevant for the moment is that reputation may not be sufficient to induce the hospital to act as if it were fully benevolent. The reason is that the effect of lower quality on reputation may well be uncertain and, in any case, loss of reputation has consequences only for the future and that may be of less concern to the hospital than the more immediate present.

But whatever the reason for partial benevolence, it enables a health authority to get better-quality services without full audit than from a purely self-interested hospital even when demand does not respond to the quality provided. However, as explained in Chalkley and Malcomson (1995b), it will typically make sense for the health authority to include some degree of cost reimbursement in the contract as long as the monitoring of actual costs is not itself too costly. The intuition is that having no cost reimbursement would provide the correct incentives to keep costs down but result in too low quality. At the margin, it is worth relaxing the incentive to keep costs down in order to achieve somewhat higher quality.

This is theory. Do hospitals actually respond to incentives in the way theory suggests? The change in the payment system for Medicare in the US in 1983 from cost reimbursement to prospective payment dramatically altered the incentives for hospitals to cut costs of treatment because with prospective payment additional costs are borne entirely by the hospital instead of being reimbursed from the Medicare budget.[2] Studies of hospital costs reviewed in Ellis and McGuire (1993) indicate that, before the change, the average cost per hospital discharge *increased* by about 2 per cent per year. In the years immediately following the change, the cost per discharge *declined* by roughly 2 per cent per year. The change in incentive system may not have been the only reason for the change in costs but the evidence is at least suggestive that it had an impact in the direction theory predicts. Hodgkin and McGuire (1994) have a fuller discussion of how the changes resulting from the introduction of prospective payment correspond to the predictions from a theoretical framework.

Bidding for contracts
Suppose a health authority selects contracts according to the principles just discussed to protect quality of service. Two natural questions are: will it achieve that quality at the lowest price by having hospitals bid for contracts, thus enhancing budgetary efficiency? and will greater competition (in the form of more bidders) enable it to fulfil its priorities more completely, thus enhancing economic efficiency?

These are difficult questions to which the literature does not provide definitive answers. When the health authority does not know the price at which the potential bidders are able to provide any given level of service, it will enhance budgetary efficiency to alter the contracts suggested in the previous section to increase the provision for payment that depends on the costs the hospital actually incurs in providing the services (or add such a provision if it is not there), as long as it is not too costly to make these costs verifiable. To see why, consider the case of a self-interested hospital with a contract that has a lump sum plus a fixed payment per patient treated. Such a contract provides a strong incentive for the hospital to keep costs to a minimum because it will retain any savings. But, if it is actually a very low-cost hospital, it will make a great deal of profit that the health authority would prefer (in line with budgetary efficiency) to use for treating other patients. Profits could be kept low by a contract that reimburses the hospital for its actual costs of treatment. This is what happens with private medical insurance and what used to happen with the cost reimbursement rules previously used for Medicare in the US. Such a contract can prevent the hospital making excessive profits but it also provides no incentive to keep costs low because any cost savings made by the hospital simply result in it being paid that much less for providing the service. The best the health authority can typically do under these circumstances is to offer a contract that specifies a maximum payment and a target cost, with the payment to the hospital reduced below the maximum by a proportion of the amount by which the actual cost falls below the target cost. With such a contract, the bidder still has an incentive to reduce costs because it receives a share of the cost savings but also, if costs turn out to be low, it does not make as large profits as with a contract that has payment independent of costs. Laffont and Tirole (1993, Chap. 1) have a detailed (but technical) discussion of the precise form the contract should take.

Use of such a contract makes bidding more complicated. The reason is that the contract has several dimensions (the maximum payment, the target cost and the share of cost reductions retained by the bidder), so selecting the winning bid is not a simple matter of choosing the lowest. Nevertheless, it is possible to design a bidding process that will select the lowest-cost bidder. Moreover, the overall cost will on average fall as the number of bidders is increased, so increased competition enhances budgetary efficiency by reducing costs. The reason is essentially the same as in the case of simple bidding discussed above – the more bidders there are, the lower on average will be the reservation price of the second lowest bidder and, hence, the price of the winning bid. For further details, see Laffont and Tirole (1993, Chap. 7).

That is not, however, the whole story because we are concerned here with what such bidding does to the quality of service provided. The conclusions just drawn apply to self-interested hospitals when demand does not respond to quality and the contract provides incentives to keep costs down. In the case in which patients correctly assess quality and their demand for treatment responds rapidly to that, we conjecture that, because quality can then be ensured by patient demand, these conclusions continue to apply. These same conclusions almost certainly also apply to hospitals that are at least partially benevolent. But there is likely to be a real problem if demand does not respond to some aspects of quality and bidders consist of some self-interested hospitals and some benevolent hospitals, with the health authority not knowing which is which. For any given contract, benevolent hospitals will provide a quality of service closer to that which the health authority would like. However, a concern that has been expressed about many public services put out to tender in the UK is that, by awarding the contract to the lowest bidder, it will go to a self-interested bidder who has no concern for the quality of service or, at the very least, successful bidders who, although they would like to provide a higher-quality service, have to settle for low quality in order to keep their prices down to the level of bidders who are unconcerned with quality. Whether this will in fact be the case and, if so, what a health authority can do about it is an issue for future research.

Quality, reputations and long term contracts
Contracts between health authorities and hospitals typically last for a year, after which a new contract is negotiated. Each contract covers the services to be provided during that year. Short-term, renewable contracts like these can give a powerful incentive for a hospital to provide a good-quality service even if patient demand does not respond to quality as long as the health authority receives some feedback on the quality of service, however informal.

For quality to be enforced by contract, it needs to be verifiable. But, at the time a new contract is awarded, a health authority can make use of any information it has, even if not verifiable, to affect either the terms of the contract it awards or which provider it is awarded to. (Unverifiable information of this type is termed *observable* in the literature.) By offering less good terms, or threatening to switch providers, if the information indicates that quality is unsatisfactory, the health authority can make it costly in the future for a hospital to skimp on quality now and thus make the hospital behave as if it were at least partially benevolent. Indeed, provided sufficient information about quality is fed back to the authority, the hospital cares sufficiently about the future (its discount rate is not too high), and future custom is sufficiently valuable, the concern for reputation can ensure that the hospital provides precisely the quality of service the health authority would like. See Gibbons (1992) for an accessible discussion of this issue. The threat to award the contract to an alternative provider becomes more powerful if there is competition among providers.

The use of short-term, renewable contracts can, however, give rise to problems. Two that have been widely discussed in the literature are the *ratchet effect* and the *hold-up effect*. The ratchet effect was first widely discussed in the literature on central planning in the former Soviet Union. The essential issue is the following. Soviet factory managers were given an output quota to fulfil. To encourage production, the factory received a bonus if it overfulfilled its quota. But, by overfulfilling the quota, the managers would reveal to the central planners that they had the capacity to produce more than their current quota. So the planners would not unnaturally seek to increase the quota the following year, with the result that the factory would have to work harder to fulfil the higher quota. So canny managers were faced with a calculation. Overfulfilling quota would result in a bonus this year but harder work (or a lower bonus) next. The effect of the planners' response to an overfulfilled quota was to reduce the incentive for higher output that the bonus was intended to provide.

The ratchet effect also arises with contract negotiation. A hospital that works hard to cut costs this year reveals that it can provide services at lower prices. A health authority that would like additional funds to spend elsewhere will then naturally bargain for lower prices next year, which reduces the incentive for the hospital to cut costs.

The hold-up effect can be illustrated as follows. Suppose a hospital can install equipment that would reduce the cost of providing services but that, once installed, could not be resold for anything like its original cost. The difference between the cost of installation and the resale value is a *sunk cost*. Under a fixed price contract, the hospital will get the cost savings that result from the installation while the contract lasts. But when it comes to negotiating the next contract, the health authority is in a position to bargain for services at lower prices because of the hospital's investment. In the extreme, if the health authority captures all the cost savings, the hospital will install equipment only if the cost savings under the *existing* contract will pay for the installation. But even if the health authority captures only a part of the cost savings, the hospital will invest too little in new equipment with consequences for both the cost and quality of service it is able to offer. The classic discussion of hold-up is in Williamson (1985). Hold-up is not just a theoretical possibility: one negotiator for an NHS trust asked us unprompted how the trust could prevent the health authority exploiting its investments in this way.

Both the ratchet effect and the hold-up effect can be alleviated by having a longer-term contract.[3] In both cases, the longer it is before the contract comes up for renewal, the more time there is for the hospital to get the benefits of its investment before the health authority captures some of those benefits in a new contract. But long-term contracts have the disadvantage of reducing the power of reputation effects because a hospital that delivers poor quality can do so for longer before losing its contract. There is thus a trade-off between having longer-term contracts to mitigate the ratchet and hold-up effects and having shorter-term contracts to maintain quality. We know of no analysis that has investigated this trade-off fully.

Conclusion

Our discussion can be summarized as follows. We envisage four potential roles for competition between suppliers: reducing the economic inefficiencies that can arise from monopoly power; reducing the influence of providers over purchasers' decisions; ensuring that services respond to what patients want; and providing information to purchasers both about which supplier can provide services for the lowest prices and how low those prices can be. The first of these does not seem very important at present in view of the countervailing bargaining power that health authorities have. It might become a serious issue if, for example, one hospital group were to buy up a chain of hospitals that formed a significant part of the UK market or if purchasers were to become sufficiently fragmented, perhaps as a result of the growth of GP fundholding. There are, however, other mechanisms for dealing with these. Indeed, a mechanism to counteract the fragmented purchasing power of GP fundholders is already developing in the form of purchasing consortia that negotiate with providers on behalf of groups of GP practices. The second potential role is one for which we know of no formal analysis. However, there are formal analyses of competition between suppliers for influence over decision-makers that suggest such competition is very wasteful and such waste must be set against any gains increased competition may have. The third may be partially addressed by increased use of GP fundholders if GPs are more closely in touch with the needs and wants of their patients than health authorities. Whether or not they are, however, is not an issue that theory can address and there is not as yet sufficient experience to provide an assessment of how this aspect of GP fundholding works in practice. The fourth role for competition may well become increasingly important as a consequence of the separation of purchasers from providers. As time goes by, those employed by health authorities are becoming more distanced from their former responsibility for the direct provision of services and may thus become less knowledgeable about the prices at which services could be provided. Increased competition between hospitals may then enhance economic efficiency and also, by enabling health authorities to get services provided at a lower cost, budgetary efficiency.

Getting hospitals to bid for contracts to provide health services is not, however, like conducting an auction for wheat because the quality (in the widest sense) of the services to be provided is not easily specified by contract. Taking the lowest bid may simply result in the provision of poor-quality services. It is here that the form of contract becomes important. Contracts must be designed carefully to ensure that the quantity and quality of services are kept as close as possible to what the health authority would like. An obvious problem is that, when quality cannot be verified, high quality will be delivered only if the hospital chooses, or is induced by the contract, to provide it. The form of contract appropriate for this depends among other things on the extent to which patients can correctly assess the quality on offer and choose where to be treated on the basis of their assessments, and also on how much the provider really cares about the interests of patients, as opposed to just its own self-interest. There is a danger in awarding a contract to the lowest bidder. Hospitals that care enough about their patients would provide the quality of service the health authority wants if given the funds to do so. But they will have to offer a low-quality service to compete with bidders who are less concerned about their patients and who therefore offer lower quality.

The key problem that we return to again here is that there are many dimensions of quality that cannot be enforced by contract. One way to alleviate this problem is to use short-term contracts that a health authority can refuse to renew if it has doubts about the quality of services that have been provided. Refusing to renew a contract does not need concrete evidence of the type that would be needed to demonstrate in court that a hospital had not fulfilled the quality terms in a contract. So a decision on renewal can make use of much more subjective assessments based on whatever information the health authority can glean. Where loss of reputation for quality results in the loss of valued future contracts, it can act as a powerful incentive to maintain standards. But the use of short-term contracts has its own problems. In particular, it can give rise to the ratchet and hold-up effects which result in services being provided at a higher cost than with a long-term contract. The trade-off between using short-term contracts to maintain quality and long-term contracts to alleviate the ratchet and hold-up effects is not easily escaped.

Our overall assessment of the current situation is as follows. There are certainly potential roles for competition in the provision of health services, though we are not convinced that the traditional anti-monopoly role is the most important. But there are also potential dangers from competition that arise from the variability in the quality of health services and the fact that quality is not easily verified (and not, therefore, easily enforced by contract). Whether or not the recent reforms in the NHS lead to better health services depends at least in part on purchasers and providers understanding what these roles and dangers are and choosing contract forms that ensure standards of quality are high. In this chapter, we have set out at least some of the issues involved.

Notes

1. In technical terminology, budgetary efficiency corresponds to the maximum of a purely utilitarian social welfare function when there is a deadweight loss to raising taxes for the health authority's budget.
2. Even under prospective payment there is some provision for reimbursing hospitals for exceptionally expensive cases but this applies to only a small proportion of cases.
3. We say *alleviated* and not *solved* advisedly. Even if the contract were to last indefinitely, the effects can occur because of circumstances in which it is in the interests of *both* parties to renegotiate the contract. A contract can always be renegotiated if both parties agree. The ratchet and hold-up effects can then occur because it is typically the case that renegotiation of an existing contract has some of the properties of negotiation of a new contract. Milgrom and Roberts (1992) provide an accessible discussion of this issue. We do not pursue it here.

References

Arrow, Kenneth J. (1963), 'Uncertainty and the welfare economics of medical care', *American Economic Review*, **53** (5), 941–69.

Barker, Kit (1993), 'NHS contracts, restitution and the internal market', *Modern Law Review*, **56** (6), 832–43.

Barker, Kit (1995), 'NHS contracting: shadows in the law of tort?', *Medical Law Review*, **3** (3), 161–76.

Binmore, Ken (1992), *Fun and Games: A Text on Game Theory*, Lexington, Mass.: D.C. Heath and Company.

Chalkley, Martin and Malcomson, James M. (1995a), 'Contracting for health services with unmonitored quality', University of Southampton, Department of Economics.

Chalkley, Martin and Malcomson, James M. (1995b), 'Contracting for health services when demand does not reflect quality', University of Southampton, Department of Economics.

Dawson, Diane (1994), 'Costs and prices in the internal market: markets vs NHS Management Executive guidelines', University of York, Centre for Health Economics, Discussion Paper 115.

Ellis, Randall P. and McGuire, Thomas G. (1993), 'Supply-side and demand-side cost sharing in health care', *Journal of Economic Perspectives*, **7** (4), 135–51.

Ferguson, Brian and Palmer, Stephen (1994), 'Markets and the NHSME guidelines: costs and prices in the NHS internal market', University of York, Centre for Health Economics, Discussion Paper 120.

Gibbons, Robert (1992), *A Primer in Game Theory*, London: Harvester Wheatsheaf.

Hodgkin, Dominic and McGuire, Thomas G. (1994), 'Payment levels and hospital response to prospective payment', *Journal of Health Economics*, **13**, 1–29.

Laffont, Jean-Jacques and Tirole, Jean (1993), *A Theory of Incentives in Procurement and Regulation*, Cambridge, Mass.: MIT Press.

Lancaster, Kelvin J. (1979), *Variety, Equity and Efficiency*, New York: Columbia University Press.

Ma, Ching-to Albert (1994), 'Health care payment systems: cost and quality incentives', *Journal of Economics and Management Strategy*, **3** (1), 93–112.

McAfee, R. Preston and McMillan, John (1987), 'Auctions and bidding', *Journal of Economic Literature*, **25** (2), 699–738.

Milgrom, Paul and Roberts, John (1992), *Economics, Organization and Management*, Englewood Cliffs, NJ: Prentice-Hall.

Myerson, Roger and Satterthwaite, Mark (1983), 'Efficient mechanisms for bilateral trading', *Journal of Economic Theory*, **28**, 265–81.

Nitzan, Shmuel (1994), 'Modelling rent-seeking contests', *European Journal of Political Economy*, **10** (1), 41–60.

Tirole, Jean (1989), *The Theory of Industrial Organization*, Cambridge, Mass.: MIT Press.

Williamson, Oliver E. (1985), *The Economic Institutions of Capitalism*, New York: The Free Press.

5 Purchasing to meet need*

Cam Donaldson

Introduction

The UK National Health Service (NHS) was established in 1948 with the dual aims of removing the price barrier to health care and eliminating the backlog of sickness in the population. The latter aim has never been achieved. Claims on health care resources continue to outstrip the availability of such resources. This problem is a global one. It is present not just in low-spending countries, such as the UK.

Without the price mechanism, however, some other mechanism is required to enable decisions to be made as to how resources can best be used. As Sheldon and Maynard (1993) have pointed out, there have been several statements by policy-makers and politicians about how resources will *not* be allocated. Two examples of such statements are as follows:

> [The NHS] imposes no limits on availability, e.g. limitation based on financial means, age, sex, employment or vocation, area of residence or insurance qualification.
>
> (Ministry of Health 1946)

> The principle that adequate health care should be provided for all, regardless of their ability to pay, must be the foundation of any arrangements for financing health care.
>
> (Margaret Thatcher, Conservative Party Conference speech, 1982)

It is relatively easy to make such statements which indicate that there will be no discrimination by age, sex or whatever. However, the more difficult issue to address is how resources *should* be allocated, an issue about which policy-makers and politicians have been uncharacteristically silent – for over 46 years!

One of the problems is that, pre-1990, it was never entirely clear who was responsible for health care priority setting. As a result of the 1990 NHS Reform and Community Care Act, responsibility for purchasing health care for communities has been placed firmly in the hands of health care purchasers, such as health authorities (health boards in Scotland) and general practi-

*The author is grateful to Gavin Mooney, Elizabeth Russell, Phil Shackley and David Torgerson for comments on an earlier draft of this paper. HERU is funded by the Chief Scientist Office of the Scottish Office Home and Health Department (SOHHD); however, the views expressed in this paper are those of the author, not SOHHD.

tioner (GP) fundholders. It is now the responsibility of health authorities to identify the needs of their populations and arrange for these needs to be met. Inevitably, this will involve such purchasers in priority setting, i.e. in deciding which needs will or will not be met and the extent to which needs will be met. However, there has still been no offer of advice on the approach to be taken or on how to go about this process. An exception to this is the Welsh Office which has offered guidance to purchasers on priority-setting, which includes the use of economics techniques (Cohen 1994).

The aim of this paper is to propose an economics approach to the priority-setting process. The arguments put forward in favour of an economics approach are not new. The language of the NHS is new, using words like 'purchasers' and 'providers'. But the economics is still about resource allocation. What is new is that the responsibilities allocated to health care purchasers now render priority-setting a task less easily avoided.

In the following section, the important distinction between health needs and health care needs is drawn. Some concepts of need, and how they can be used in health care priority setting, are then outlined. It will be argued that the economics concept is the one more likely to lead to maximization of benefits to the community with available resources. A case study on implementing the economics approach is then outlined. Other practical considerations will also be addressed. These include discussions of the role of GP fundholders in purchasing to meet needs, whether and how equity criteria can be used in such purchasing, and whether, from an economics perspective, there is a role for the consumer in health care purchasing.

Health needs versus need for health care

Health care needs and health needs are not the same thing. Health care is instrumental in the promotion and (it is hoped) the achievement of better health. There are, however, several other instruments for achieving improvements in health. These include better education, improved housing, other environmental improvements and changes in personal behaviour, such as eating habits. Thus, the alleviation of a health need may require any one (or combination) of several instruments or agencies.

Therefore, although it is perfectly reasonable for health care purchasers to advocate that *health* needs be better met, it may not be within their powers to purchase services to allow this to happen. In the UK, better hygiene and housing, for instance, are responsibilities of other bodies. *Health care* needs are those which can be met only by the utilization of health care.

The distinction between health and health care needs is important for practical as well as academic reasons. Even though health care purchasers may think that health needs are important, it is ultimately health *care* needs among which health care purchasers have to prioritize. Therefore, in this paper, discussion will be limited to needs which can be addressed by the purchase of health care, i.e. 'health care needs'.

Purchasing to meet health care needs

The concept of need
There are several notions of health care need. Not all are helpful for priority setting. Bradshaw (1972) defined four types of need. They are as follows:

1. *Normative need* is a third party's (usually an expert's) definition of need. It could be based on an explicit or implicit standard. If a person falls below that standard s/he is defined as being 'in need'. This definition is useful in highlighting two things. First, need is a matter of opinion. Second, given this, it is not surprising that views of need vary so much. This could be one explanation for the existence of variations in medical practice within and between countries (Andersen and Mooney 1990).
2. *Felt need* can be equated with want. It is a need felt by the individual. Individuals' perceptions of need may not conform to the perceptions of society. To take an extreme example, the statement 'I need a Rolls Royce' would be treated differently by society than would the statement 'I need a plaster cast for my broken leg'. So, once again, what society does in response to such felt needs depends on a third party and, therefore, opinion. The example of Rolls Royces and broken legs is used simply to show that people would respond differently to the word 'need' used in different contexts. In fact there would (it is hoped!) be little disagreement about which of these represents a more genuine need. However, more controversy would be likely to arise in cases such as *in-vitro* fertilization and grommet insertion. Do these represent health care needs?
3. *Expressed need* is a felt need turned into action (i.e. when a want becomes a demand on services). For instance, the most common form of expressed need for health care is when a person visits her/his GP. This demand is determined by individuals' perceptions of the benefits of consultation as well as time and monetary costs. Once again, however, the third party (in this case the GP) is called upon to confirm or dispel such a demand as a need.
4. *Comparative need* involves comparing those in receipt of a service with those not in such receipt. If those not in receipt have the same characteristics as those who are in receipt, then, according to at least some concepts of fairness or justice, the former should be given the service too.

These classifications of need are useful in highlighting that need is value-laden (i.e. a matter of opinion) and that there is no reason to believe that society's response to the same need expressed at different times and in different parts of the country will be uniform.

Probably the least helpful of Bradshaw's definitions is the fourth one. It represents an ideal which may not be achievable due to resource constraints. But if it is interpreted in terms of equity, it will have to be recognized that to allow equal access to (or use of) services for equal need will result in resources being taken from some other beneficial use. This is where the role of economics comes in, as expressed in the classic works of Williams (1974) and Culyer (1976). Their insights may sound simple twenty years later, but still remain unrecognized by many and are, in fact, the key to allocating resources in health care. The crucial point they make is that a need for one item is not independent of the need for another. This is because meeting a need involves the use of some of society's scarce resources. The opportunity to use these resources in meeting another need is forgone, i.e. there is an opportunity 'cost' in meeting any need. Therefore, in order to maximize the amount of need met by our limited pot of (health care) resources it is necessary to know the amount of need that is met by an intervention (i.e. *marginal met need*) and the amount of resources used in meeting this need (i.e. the cost). Only by combining the cost of interventions with the marginal met need of each can we choose the combination of services which maximizes the amount of need met overall.

The concept of marginal met need represents a breakthrough in that it is the only concept of need which is usable in a world of scarce resources. This concept of need is embedded in the notion of positive marginal productivity. If a health care intervention (as judged by a third party, like a doctor) could be of benefit to an individual, then that individual is said to have 'ability to benefit' and is in need. If the resources would do no good (i.e. produce no benefit), how can a person be in need? The requirement, then, is to measure ability to benefit; that is, measure the increases in benefit that could be brought about by different types of health care. Once this is matched with costs, the combination of health care interventions can be chosen which maximizes benefit (or met need) in the community.

To complete the argument, it is also important to discuss what is meant by benefit. The usual way of conceptualizing the benefits of health care is in terms of health improvements (recently referred to as health gain). Indeed, this would seem to be the main benefit from such care. The author prefers a classification reflecting broader aspects of the utility derived from health care. This could include such aspects as information (from screening) and autonomy (in long-term care for elderly people). The danger of such a broad definition is that it becomes too broad, with 'illegitimate' aspects of benefit, such as utility from having television sets at the end of the bed, receiving too much prominence (or, indeed, any prominence at all). However, what the author has in mind are broader aspects of utility which are integral to the health care on offer. Autonomy and TV sets may be seen as integral to long-term care, but not to acute or elective surgery. One further point is that some health economists may argue that it is possible to define all the broader aspects of utility as *health* effects. For example, provision of information and greater autonomy could be said to affect mental health. The danger with this, however, is one of reducing all economics to *health* economics!

Using 'need' in health care purchasing
There are three main approaches to using the concept of ability to benefit in health care purchasing. The first is the Thatcher approach (see the quotation on p. 88) of 'health care for all'. Once an ability to benefit (i.e. a need) has been recognized, it must be met. Generous though it may seem, this approach is unhelpful for health care purchasing. Purchasers, faced with limited funds, cannot meet all needs. The problem, then, is how best to allocate resources. One way of doing this is to attempt to produce the most benefit (met need) possible (a point to which we shall return in this subsection).

The second approach is the 'burden-of-illness' approach to priority setting. Proponents of this approach would measure the total amount of ill health, categorized by disease, and claim that this gives a picture of relative 'need'. Priorities are then set according to the size of the need. Priority, in terms of use of health care resources, would then go to alleviating or analysing the diseases which are the big killers, big resource users or big causers of morbidity in society. Other similar burden-of-illness approaches to priority setting are 'cost-of-illness' studies (Shiell et al. 1987). The most prominent examples in UK health care policy-making are the uses of this approach in the documents *The Health of the Nation* and *Scotland's Health* (Secretary of State for Health 1991; Scottish Office, 1992a).

Such approaches simply tell us whether one problem is bigger than another. For priority setting, they do not actually come up with a resource allocation rule except to say 'the bigger the problem the more money it should get'. Except by chance, this rule is unlikely to lead to the objective of maximizing benefits to the community given resource constraints. There are two major flaws with such an approach. These stem directly from the economics approach to need introduced in the previous subsection. First, 'total need' *per se* is a red herring. It is changes in need (or marginal met need) that should constitute the outcome measure. It is not the size of a disease or illness that counts but what can be done about it in terms of the effectiveness of interventions. The effectiveness of an intervention constitutes the marginal need met by that intervention. The second flaw is that changes in costs resulting from interventions are ignored. Meeting more of one need has an opportunity cost in that less of other needs will be met. This can be seen immediately if we pose the question: if the cost of heart transplants fell to 1 per cent of their current cost, would the priority attached to heart transplants change? (Clue: need has not changed, but the cost of meeting it has.)

Remember, it is only by matching the costs of health care interventions to the benefits produced that we can choose the mix of health care resources which maximizes benefit (or met need) to the community. This does not mean, however, that economists would propose to measure the costs and benefits of all existing and new health care. Given that every health board or authority already has a given starting point in terms of its current uses of resources, the important thing is to make *changes* in such allocations which result in greater benefit than before. Thus, we need only analyse the costs and benefits of the proposed changes. Economists call such analysis 'marginal analysis'. It should be borne in mind at this stage, that despite the everyday-language association of the word 'marginal' with 'insignificant', in health economics it is a crucial concept. It focuses on change, and, within the context of health care purchasing, such change can be large or small. The danger of being unaware of marginal analysis is that the alternative is to focus on the average. However, when expanding or reducing a service, for instance, costs do not change in accordance with the average.

A common example which is used to demonstrate the different results from the use of the economics approach as opposed to a burden-of-illness approach is chiropody for elderly people. This has been shown to represent good value for money in terms of health gains relative to resources spent (Bryan et al. 1991). Yet, it would not rank highly under a burden-of-illness approach, as, relative to other conditions, foot problems do not cause major morbidity or mortality or lead to large health care costs in total.

The principles supporting an economics approach may seem straightforward. However, the application of such an approach is not so straightforward. It is this issue of the application of an economics approach to which we now turn.

Purchasing to meet need: implementing the economics approach

To illustrate the economics approach to purchasing to meet need, consider the alternatives for a programme aimed at reducing heart disease amongst a population of 200,000 males aged 40–49 (Kristiansen et al. 1991). One alternative is to promote healthy eating in the population *in combination with* GP screening for high cholesterol levels (serum concentration 6.0–7.9 mmol/l) followed by dietary treatment for those in the relevant range. This we will refer to as the *combined approach*. (In the paper referenced, drug treatment was implemented for those with serum cholesterol above 8 mmol/l. This alternative is not considered here.) An alternative is to use population promotion of healthy eating on its own. This we will refer to as the *population approach*.

It is assumed that health gain is measured in terms of 'healthy years'. Years of life in states of less than 'full health' (e.g. disability) are still important, and can be converted to healthy years by the use of various techniques. To date, the most common form of conversion is quality-adjusted life years (QALYs), although another technique, healthy years equivalents (HYEs) is gaining favour (Williams 1985; Torrance 1986; Mehrez and Gafni 1989; Gafni and Zylak 1990). The relative merits of QALYs and HYEs have been discussed by Culyer and Wagstaff (1993) and Gafni and Birch (1993).

Referring to the third row of data in Table 5.1, the total cost of the combined approach has been estimated at about £40,038,000 with a total benefit of 4,200 healthy years. This gives an average cost of £9,530 per healthy year gained. Whether this represents a reasonable investment is open to question. However, the question is put beyond doubt when examining marginal costs. The second row of data reveals that the population approach alone would have yielded 3,800 healthy years anyway, at a cost of £38,000, or £10 per healthy year gained. The additional 400 healthy years are gained by the combined approach at an additional cost of £40m – a marginal cost of £100,000 per healthy year gained. The marginal cost per healthy year gained by the combined programme is over ten times its average cost (thus highlighting the danger of looking at simple averages and, hence, the importance of marginal analysis!). Referring to the description of the margin above, a reorientation of health care resources to permit the addition of screening and dietary treatment would presumably be judged as not worthwhile. The opportunity cost is too great, or, in plainer language, the resources could be better spent on some other activity which would make a greater contribution to reducing need or to health production.

A sharper distinction between average and marginal costs is displayed in a study by Neuhauser and Lewicki (1976). They examined the recommendation by the American Cancer Society that six sequential tests of stool be carried out in order to test for cancer of the colon. The average cost per case detected after the sixth test was $2,145 (i.e. $176,337÷71.942). However, the incremental gain from carrying out six tests instead of five was very small (rising from 71.9417 to 71.9420 cases detected in a population of 10,000, 72 of whom are estimated to have the condition). The incremental cost of carrying out six tests instead of five was $13,190. Therefore, the marginal cost per case detected in moving from five to six tests was $47,107,214 (i.e. $13,190÷0.0003). The study showed that it may not be worth going beyond two or three tests. Note also that the study does not provide an exact answer to the question of how many tests are worthwhile. It is for policy-makers (purchasers?) to decide what an extra case of cancer detected is worth. Although an exact answer is not provided by the economics in this case, we

Table 5.1 Costs and benefits of strategies to reduce cholesterol

Strategy	(1) Total cost (£)	(2) Total benefit (Healthy years)	(3) Added cost (£)	(4) Added benefit (Healthy years)	(5) Average cost per healthy year [(1)–(2)]	(6) Marginal cost per healthy year [(3)–(4)]
No action	0	0	0	0	–	–
Population	38,000	3,800	38,000	3,800	£10	£10
Combined	40,038,000	4,200	40,000,000	400	£9,530	£100,000

Source: Kristiansen et al. (1991).

95

do end up with a more efficient solution than if the decision had been taken in the absence of economic analysis.

Returning to the example of cholesterol screening in Table 5.1, the example used is based on data from a study carried out in Norway (Kristiansen et al. 1991). The study is useful for demonstrating the principles of an economics approach and for demonstrating data requirements for economic evaluations of such activities. The data used by the authors of the study are listed in Table 5.2. Estimation of resource consequences is relatively straightforward in this case. However, this is not so with elicitation of data for estimating benefits (some of which have implications for estimating costs averted). Epidemiological data were used to make the links between: the programmes and effects on cholesterol levels; reduced cholesterol levels and effects on infarctions; and reduced infarctions and effects on mortality and life years saved. Estimates of effects on quality of life relied on assumptions made by the authors. For instance, it was estimated that being labelled 'at risk' would result in a 0.2 per cent reduction in quality of life for one's remaining life years.

Table 5.2   Estimating benefits and costs of strategies to reduce cholesterol

---

Data required on resources used in the following:
  Screening
  Confirmatory screening test
  Doctor visits
  Cholesterol testing
  Treatment of coronary heart disease
  Coronary artery bypass grafting
  Treatment after infarction
  Population strategy

Data required for estimation of benefits (and averted costs):
  Effect of programmes on lowering cholesterol
  Effect of reducing cholesterol on heart disease and, therefore, myocardial
    infarctions
  How many of these infarctions would have been fatal?
  Fatalities need to be age specific so as to work out life years saved
  Quality of life:
    – of being identified as 'at risk'
    – improvement associated with avoiding a non-fatal infarction
    – improvement associated with a fatal infarction avoided!

It can be seen from this example that implementing the economics approach is not simple. Many data are required. What is important is to measure benefits of candidates for more and less resources in the best terms possible. Getting the best data on costs and outcomes of possible changes puts the purchaser in the best position for judging which service reductions or expansions should go ahead so that more need can be met in total. More often than not, however, there are no such data on QALYs or other measures of health outcome which relate to local issues to be addressed by purchasers. We are a long way from outcome-based change in the NHS.

However, even though the practical difficulties may seem sizeable, it should be remembered that the most important thing about the economics approach is the *framework* it provides – a framework for organizing information and a framework for thinking with regard to priority setting for purchasing. In many priority-setting situations, the best one can hope for is simply a *description* of the possible outcomes of each option assessed. Indeed this should be a minimum requirement. If health care providers cannot even provide (admittedly biased!) descriptions of the benefits of their activities, should they really be doing them at all? If such descriptions can be supplied, intangible costs and benefits can then be considered alongside those which are more readily measurable. The trade-offs between such benefits and costs will still be explicit. It is the author's contention that 'even crude estimates of costs and benefits, representing conditions prevailing in a local context, would serve priority setting better than attempting accurate measurement of the wrong thing' (Donaldson and Farrar 1993).

Outstanding issues
Up to now, this paper has addressed the issue of how health authorities can go about the process of purchasing so as to maximize the amount of need met with their resources. Issues which also need to be addressed are whether GPs can purchase in a similar way, the role of considerations of equity in the economics approach and whether there is a role for consumers within such a framework.

Whither GP fundholding?
As well as providing primary health care, GPs can elect to have their own budgets for the purchase of a narrow range of services. Some of the funds for these budgets are deducted from allocations to health authorities. The range of services which can be purchased from such budgets include elective in-patient referrals (up to a cumulative cost of £5,000 per person), outpatient visits (except antenatal and obstetrics), and community health services (such as district nursing and health visiting) which have to be purchased from an NHS provider. The remainder of the funds come from Family Health Service

Authorities and cover prescribing, a proportion of practice staff costs and practice management and computing costs. Virement across headings is permitted, except for the community health services allocation.

In principle, there is no reason why fundholders could not use the economics techniques outlined above in their priority-setting process. There are some practical problems, however. A reasonably sized population base is required to prevent random yearly fluctuations in the need for services (Crump et al. 1991; Ratcliffe 1993). Partly as a result of this, more fundholders are coming together in consortia to make decisions while non-fundholders are working more closely with health authorities (Smith et al. 1993). However, while there is evidence of the growing use of economics techniques in health authority purchasing (Donaldson and Farrar 1993; Cohen 1994), this is not the case in general practice. Only now are GPs being exposed to the *principles* of the economics approach (Donaldson and Ratcliffe 1994).

Despite these points, it could be argued that GPs should be more receptive to economic principles and techniques. This is because they have a longer history than other doctors of being aware of resource constraints, and, in acting as an 'agent' on behalf of their patients, they are more aware of the need to make choices and, therefore, to weigh up the costs and benefits of alternative courses of action.

Although the issue of equity will be dealt with in more detail in the following subsection, it requires particular attention in the case of fundholding. In the pre-reform NHS, resources were allocated to health authorities through the RAWP (Resource Allocation Working Party) formula. This formula allocated funds on the basis of 'needs' as indicated by the age, sex and health of health authority populations. Thus, the intention was to allocate funds with the objective of providing equal access to health care for equal needs. Success was limited (Maynard and Ludbrook 1980). However, it is thought that fundholding may be even more detrimental to the objective of equity, with contracts being struck to give patients of fundholders priority in terms of treatment (Donaldson and Mooney 1993).

The role of equity in the economic approach
The role of equity in purchasing to meet need is ambiguous. This is largely because of the lack of a precise definition of health care policy with regard to equity. Equal access for equal need is one definition. There are others, however, such as 'equal utilization of health care for equal need' and 'equal health'. These definitions are not the same, and, more importantly, pursuit of one is likely to lead to different policy prescriptions from pursuit of another (Wagstaff et al. 1991; Mooney et al. 1991; Mooney 1992).

Despite this confusion, economics is, at the very least, useful in identifying *who* receives benefits and incurs cost. It is then left to purchasers to decide how to use such information. However, it is possible to imagine a situation in which maximization of met need will not be pursued because it is judged to be inequitable. Likewise, some equity may occasionally be sacrificed in order to improve efficiency.

Take the example of breast cancer screening. The objective of achieving maximum compliance in the target group of 50–64-year-old women can be interpreted as an equity objective – that of equal utilization for equal need. All women in this age group are defined as 'in equal need' and the aim is to get them to use the breast screening service. Currently, it is UK government policy to maximize compliance through the use of a fixed appointment system (Department of Health Advisory Committee 1990). With such a system, the letter of invitation includes a set date and time for the screening test to take place. The recommendation to use fixed appointments for breast screening is based on this method achieving a 10 per cent higher level of compliance than an alternative (the open appointment system) (Williams and Vessey 1989). The open appointment system is one in which the onus is on recipients to contact the screening service to arrange an appointment.

Table 5.3 Methods of recruitment for breast cancer screening

		Invitation type:		
	Fixed	Open (using data from trial)	Open (assuming target population of 188)	Open (extended target population)
No. of women invited	188	204	188	241
No. screened	162 (86%)	154 (76%)	143 (76%)	183 (76%)

The implications of the pursuit of such a policy in terms of benefits forgone has been analysed by Torgerson and Donaldson (1994) using the results from the Williams and Vessey trial which are displayed in Table 5.3. It can be seen that, if the target population is assumed to be 188 women, then only 143 (i.e. 76 per cent) would have been screened had the open invitation system been used. This compares with 162 women screened using the fixed appointment system. The fixed appointment system better meets the objective of equal utilization for equal need by improving compliance by 19 women. Yet, with the fixed appointment system, 16 appointment slots remain unused. These cannot be reallocated to other women. However, with the open appointment system, unused appointment slots *can* be reallocated. Therefore, if the target population were extended, 183 women could be screened. This increases the number of women screened using the open appointment system by 40 (i.e. 183–143).

These 40 additional women screened under the open appointment system are from a different target population from that initially envisaged. The real opportunity cost of increasing compliance in the original population by 19 women is the screening opportunity forgone by the 40 women from the extended population. The question which now arises, in efficiency terms, is whether the health benefits accruing to the 19 women outweigh those that would accrue to the 40 women from the extended population. There is some evidence that the health gain in the latter group would be greater if an older group were targeted in addition to the current group. If so, the pursuit of maximum compliance could be said to have an opportunity cost, in terms of health gain forgone, which is greater than the health gain achieved. Therefore, even without an explicit equity policy objective, it is important that purchasers know not only the magnitude of costs and benefits but also how they are distributed.

Is there a role for the consumer?

The economic arguments for extensive government intervention in health care, of which a national health service is an example, are complex. However, one of the reasons expounded for such intervention is that there is an asymmetry of information between health care consumers and suppliers of such care (Evans 1984; Donaldson and Gerard 1993). Those who supply care are the very people to whom consumers go for advice. This raises the possibility for exploitation and, along with other reasons, provides a case for extensive intervention to 'protect' consumers. The establishment of bureaucratic health care systems has thus meant that, in the past, consumers have tended to be excluded from the health care priority-setting process.

Yet, the new NHS was sold partly on the basis of increased consumer involvement (Secretaries of State for Health 1989). This is somewhat paradoxical in the light of the arguments presented in the previous paragraph. Indeed, within the current framework of health care purchasing and providing in the UK NHS there is little or no incentive to involve the consumer. The asymmetry of information that exists between patients and doctors has been little affected by the market structure. Indeed, through the implementation of fundholding in general practice, it could be argued that the position of the GP as the agent of the consumer has been strengthened. However, it is not clear whether this would lead to more or less consumer involvement in health care priority setting. Furthermore, there is the *a priori* question of whether members of the population wish to act as 'good consumers' when it comes to health care. The small amount of evidence there is indicates not, and that a push to greater involvement could penalize those less likely to want to act as consumers in the traditional sense, e.g. older people (Donaldson et al. 1991; Lupton et al. 1991).

At the collective level, it seems that the only way to ensure consumer involvement in priority setting is to regulate purchasers. Tentative moves have been made to push purchasers to take more account of consumers' views (NHS Management Executive 1992; Scottish Office 1992b). However, the form of consumer involvement is still unclear. At the moment, such surveys are more at the level of assessing patient satisfaction with services rather than eliciting their preferences with regard to alternative uses of a limited pot of resources. There is nothing wrong with this, except that the comparative advantage of the economist is not in designing and administering surveys of satisfaction. Therefore, the role of economics in eliciting consumer values may turn out to be limited either by the limited role of the consumer or because consumers' own values of such involvement are low.

Conclusion

Economics presents the only practical method for purchasing to meet need. It takes account of scarcity of resources and, therefore, the need to make choices. This does not mean that economists would propose evaluation of the costs and benefits of every health care activity. Indeed, by recommending marginal analysis, economists recognize the reality of incremental change in the health service, i.e. that more often than not it is about having a balance of care and altering that balance to meet more need rather than getting rid of or introducing whole new services.

In purchasing within the context of primary care, there is no reason why economics techniques cannot be used. Many practical issues remain to be resolved. However, if they can be overcome, the use of economics in this setting, combined with its increased use at the health authority level, should ensure more equitable and efficient health care purchasing.

With regard to equity, it is at least possible to use economics techniques to examine who receives the benefits and who bears the costs of any health care purchasing decision. This also makes it clear whether any such decision will actually result in less total benefit to the community as a result of a more equitable distribution of such benefits. The role of economics in eliciting consumers' values is currently limited. It is unclear whether this will remain the case in the future.

Finally, we come full circle, back to the Welsh affinity with priority-setting. In this respect, it is interesting to note that even the so-called 'idealist', Aneurin Bevan, at least recognized scarcity of resources. In defending the National Health Service Bill in committee stage, he said, in response to a proposal to make domestic help and some related services free of financial charge,

Our objection to the means' test was that it was devised for the purpose of withholding money from people. This means' test is for the purpose of giving services to people who are in need of these services ... and where people can make a contribution towards the cost, they should make it. (House of Commons 1946)

Whether or not one agrees with the proposed remedy of charging for such services, the point is that there is a cost to meeting need. One can speculate, if I had mistakenly attributed this quotation to Thatcher and Thatcher's to Bevan, if any readers would have noticed. Until reading the above quotation in an article by Maynard (1980), I would not have!

References

Andersen, T.F. and Mooney, G. (eds) (1990), *The Challenges of Medical Practice Variations*, London: Macmillan.

Bradshaw, J. (1972), 'The concept of social need', *New Society*, 640–43, March.

Bryan, S., Parkin, D. and Donaldson, C. (1991), 'Chiropody and the QALY: a case study in assigning categories of disability and distress to patients', *Health Policy*, **18**, 169–85.

Cohen, D. (1994), 'Marginal analysis in practice: an alternative to needs assessment in the allocation of health care resources', *British Medical Journal*, **309**, 781–4.

Crump, B.J., Cubbon, J.E., Drummond, M.F., Hawkes, R.A. and Marchment, M.D. (1991), 'Fundholding in general practice and financial risk', *British Medical Journal*, **302**, 1582–4.

Culyer, A.J. (1976), *Need and the National Health Service: Economics and Social Choice*, London: Martin Robertson.

Culyer, A.J. and Wagstaff, A. (1993), 'QALYs versus HYEs', *Journal of Health Economics*, **12**, 311–23.

Department of Health Advisory Committee (1990), *Consolidated Guidance on Breast Cancer Screening*, Oxford: Screening Publications.

Donaldson, C. and Farrar, S. (1993), 'Needs assessment: developing an economic approach', *Health Policy*, **25**, 95–108.

Donaldson, C. and Gerard, K. (1993), *Economics of Health Care Financing: the Visible Hand*, London: Macmillan.

Donaldson, C. and Mooney, G. (1993), 'The new NHS in a global context: is it taking us where we want to be?', *Health Policy*, **25**, 9–24.

Donaldson, C. and Ratcliffe, J. (1994), 'Economics and priority setting in the new NHS', *Update*, 735–36, May.

Donaldson, C., Lloyd, P. and Lupton, D. (1991), 'Primary health care consumerism amongst elderly Australians', *Age and Ageing*, **20**, 280–86.

Evans, R.G. (1984), *Strained Mercy: the Economics of Canadian Health Care*, Toronto, Butterworths.

Gafni, A. and Birch, S. (1993), 'Economics, health and health economics: HYEs versus QALYs', *Journal of Health Economics*, **11**, 325–39.

Gafni, A. and Zylak, C.J. (1990), 'Ionic versus non-ionic contrast media: a burden or a bargain?', *Canadian Medical Association Journal*, **143**, 475–8.

House of Commons (1946), *Committee Stage of the National Health Service Bill*, cols 1561–2, 18 June.

Kristiansen, I.S., Eggen, A.E. and Thelle, D.S. (1991), 'Cost effectiveness of incremental programmes for lowering serum cholesterol concentration: is individual intervention worthwhile?', *British Medical Journal*, **302**, 1119–22.

Lupton, D., Donaldson, C. and Lloyd, P. (1991), 'Caveat emptor or blissful ignorance? Patients and the consumerist ethos', *Social Science and Medicine*, **33**, 559–68.

Maynard, A. (1980), 'Medical care and the price mechanism', in Judge, K. (ed.) *Pricing the Social Services*, London: Macmillan.

Maynard, A. and Ludbrook, A. (1980), 'Budget allocation in the National Health Service', *Journal of Social Policy*, 289–312, July.

Mehrez, A. and Gafni, A. (1989), 'Quality adjusted life years, utility theory and healthy years equivalents', *Medical Decision Making*, 9, 142–9.

Mooney, G. (1992), *Economics, Medicine and Health Care* (2nd edition), Hemel Hempstead: Harvester Wheatsheaf.

Mooney, G., Hall, J., Donaldson, C. and Gerard, K. (1991), 'Utilisation as a measure of equity: weighing heat?', *Journal of Health Economics*, 10, 475–80.

Neuhauser, D. and Lewicki, A.M. (1976), 'What do we gain from the sixth stool guide?', *New England Journal of Medicine*, 293, 255–8.

NHS Management Executive (1992), *Local voices. The views of local people in purchasing for health*, London: NHSME.

Ratcliffe, J. (1993), 'Extra-market incentives in the new NHS', *Health Policy*, 25, 169–83.

Scottish Office (1992a), *Scotland's Health: a Challenge to us All*, Edinburgh: HMSO.

Scottish Office (1992b), *The patient's charter: what users think*, Edinburgh: HMSO.

Secretary of State for Health (1991), *The Health of the Nation: a Consultative Document for Health in England*, London: HMSO.

Secretaries of State for Health, Wales, Northern Ireland and Scotland (1989), *Working for Patients*, London: HMSO.

Sheldon, T.A. and Maynard, A. (1993), 'Is rationing inevitable?' In *Rationing in Action*, London: BMJ Books.

Shiell, A., Gerard, K. and Donaldson, C. (1987), 'Cost of illness studies: an aid to decision-making?' *Health Policy*, 8, 317–22.

Smith, R., Crawford, M. and Roberts, H. (1993), 'Purchasing in Practice', *Health Service Journal*, 103.

Torgerson, D and Donaldson, C (1994), 'An economic view of high compliance as a screening objective', *British Medical Journal*, 308, 117–19.

Torrance, G.W. (1986), 'Measurement of health state utilities for economic appraisal', *Journal of Health Economics*, 5, 1–30.

Wagstaff, A., van Doorslaer, E. and Paci, P. (1991), 'On the measurement of horizontal equity in the delivery of health care', *Journal of Health Economics*, 10, 169–205.

Williams, A. (1974), 'Need as a demand concept (with special reference to health)', in Culyer, A.J. (ed.) *Economic Policies and Social Goals*, London: Martin Robertson.

Williams, A. (1985), 'Economics of coronary artery bypass grafting', *British Medical Journal*, 291, 326–9.

Williams, E.M.I. and Vessey, M.P. (1989), 'Randomised trial of two strategies offering women mobile screening for breast cancer', *British Medical Journal*, 299, 158–9.

6 Capital and labour markets for health

David Mayston

Introduction

One of the most important features of the National Health Service, like other health care systems around the world, is that it is *labour-intensive* in its inputs. The total labour costs of the main Hospital and Community Health Services (HCHS) branch of the NHS account for some 64.9 per cent of total annual expenditure. Of these labour costs, expenditure on nurses and mid-wives accounts for some 45.9 per cent of the total. The impact of the NHS reforms, or any extension of these reforms, on labour costs is therefore of critical importance.

The labour-intensive nature of the NHS is in turn associated with a major source of long-term cost pressure on the NHS. This is the *relative price effect*, which arises from the tendency over time for the price of labour to rise relative to the prices of other goods, as real earnings increase over time with economic growth. While economic growth and technological progress reduce the cost of many manufactured goods, such as transistor radios, relative to consumer incomes, those commodities, such as health care, which have a high labour content, tend instead to increase in their price relative to those of other commodities, as real wages rise. In other words, the other side of the coin of rising real incomes over time is an increasing cost of labour-intensive services, such as health care, relative to the cost of other commodities in the economy.

The relative price effect can be seen in Figure 6.1. The higher curve in Figure 6.1 shows the specific pay and prices index for the main HCHS branch of the NHS. This index reflects changes in the cost of the specific items, including drugs and health care labour, which the NHS actually purchases. Labour costs are again by far the largest element of these costs. The lower curve in Figure 6.1 shows the general price level of all commodities in the UK economy, as reflected in the general GDP deflator. Mainly because of the relative price effect, the specific pay and prices index, including labour costs, has been growing more rapidly than prices in general, as Figure 6.1 confirms.

Figure 6.2 shows the effect of deflating the monetary increase in the funding of the main HCHS branch of the NHS since 1978/9 by the specific pay and prices index for the NHS. The effect of such deflation in Figure 6.2 is to show a slower rate of growth in 'real' funding in the lower dotted curve of Figure 6.1 than either the growth in monetary funding or the growth of

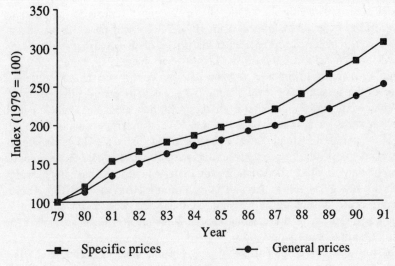

Source: DoH (1994).

Figure 6.1   General and NHS-specific price changes (1979 = 100)

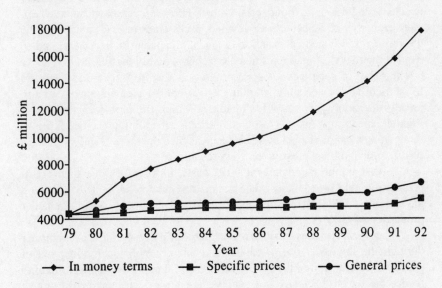

Source: DoH (1994).

Figure 6.2   NHS HCHS current expenditure in money and real terms

expenditure deflated by the GDP deflator. Largely because of the relative price effect, expenditure on the main HCHS branch of the NHS has been growing in real terms (compared to the prices of the inputs that the NHS actually purchases) at only 1.8 per cent a year since 1979, compared to a monetary increase in funding of some 11.3 per cent a year and an increase ahead of the general price level of some 3.1 per cent a year over this period.

When we turn to capital inputs into the NHS, new annual capital expenditure (on items such as new hospitals and CAT scanners) accounts for only some 7.6 per cent of total annual expenditure on the NHS. However, while new capital expenditure is a comparatively small part of total NHS expenditure, the way in which the existing capital stock is utilized has a significant effect on energy, maintenance and other running costs to the NHS. These revenue costs of running the existing capital stock account for some £1.3 billion per year, with the existing capital stock itself valued at some £25 billion (Audit Commission 1991a).

Existing capital equipment, such as X-ray machines and computer systems, is also subject to an increasing rate of *technological obsolescence* and need for *replacement expenditure*. In manufacturing industry, capital equipment is typically a substitute for labour, enabling total costs to be reduced as more productive technological advances are incorporated into new machinery to substitute for rising labour costs. In the NHS, however, new capital equipment embodying recent technological advances tends instead to increase the detection rate of medical conditions that are capable of treatment, and to expand the range of treatments that are technologically feasible.

The result of such technological progress is then to *increase* the demand for skilled labour, both to operate the more sophisticated equipment, and to process the additional cases for treatment which the new scanners detect. Capital expenditure, and the resultant demands for additional labour expenditure that new capital expenditure sets up, can also therefore readily become a further source of cost pressure on NHS resources.

A further important feature of NHS costs, however, is that they are at present low relative to many other countries, as shown in Table 6.1. Among the 24 listed OECD countries, only Turkey and Greece spend a smaller proportion of GDP on health care.

We can then ask: how much scope is there for reducing these costs further through the improved use of capital and labour? Will the introduction of greater competition into the supply of labour and capital to the NHS help to reduce these costs? Equally, however, we need to ask: are there risks of cost escalation and reducing quality of health care from making ill-considered changes to the NHS? To investigate these questions, we shall first identify a number of directions in which improved efficiency involving the use of labour and capital resources in the NHS might be achievable.

Table 6.1   *Percentage of GDP spent on health care in 1991*

Australia	8.6	Japan	6.6
Austria	8.4	Luxembourg	7.2
Belgium	7.9	Netherlands	8.4
Canada	10.0	New Zealand	7.5
Denmark	6.6	Norway	7.5
Finland	8.9	Portugal	6.7
France	9.1	Spain	6.7
Germany	8.5	Sweden	8.7
Greece	5.2	Switzerland	7.9
Iceland	8.4	Turkey	4.0
Ireland	7.3	United Kingdom	6.6
Italy	8.3	United States	13.4

Source: OECD (1993).

Possible sources of efficiency gain in the NHS

In discussing efficiency in the NHS, we may first distinguish between questions of *efficiency* in meeting any given target set of health care demands for the NHS from questions of *effectiveness* in selecting that target set. Given the doubtful or unknown effectiveness of many medical treatments in achieving improvements in the health status of patients, one main source of improved value for money in the NHS may well be to target more closely those treatments that are genuinely effective.

However, effectiveness is here a question chiefly for purchasers. Issues of efficiency, of how to deliver a given selected package of health care at minimum resource cost, intimately involve providers and the use of the key inputs of labour and capital. Nevertheless questions of both effectiveness and efficiency must ultimately be brought together, so that purchasing decisions are informed by data both on the *benefits* and clinical effectiveness of different treatments and on the *resource costs* involved when these treatments are provided in the most efficient and cost-effective way.

When we turn to ways in which labour and capital resources might be more efficiently employed in the NHS, there are a number of aspects which merit closer examination.

The first of these is the greater use of day surgery. This means that the patient has to spend less time recovering from the surgical operation in hospital, and thus potentially reduces the demands on capital and labour in the form of beds and nursing care. Increases in the number of day cases have been a main source of increases in labour productivity that offset to some extent the above relative price effect. The Audit Commission (1990, p. 5) estimated that 'if all DHAs [district health authorities] performed day surgery consistently at readily achievable levels for each of 20 common procedures, an additional 186,000 patients could be treated without increased expenditure'. The Audit Commission also considered that 'many other procedures are suitable for day surgery, offering potential for 300,000 additional patients to be treated annually', and equivalent to about 34 per cent of the existing waiting lists for day cases and inpatients in England and Wales.

However, the Audit Commission (1990, p. 19) then stated that

> Day-case performance is difficult to assess because the available data often lack sufficient detail and are not consistent from one health authority to another. Without a clear assessment of the current position it is impossible to estimate the likely potential for expansion and to draw up plans for achieving it.

The scope for resource saving from the wider introduction of day surgery is likely to be limited by the following considerations:

1. Day surgery involves a saving at marginal cost of relatively cheap recovery time compared to the more expensive cost of the operation itself.
2. Day cases may require more experienced and more expensive medical staff, such as consultants rather than junior doctors (Bryan 1995).
3. Day cases may require an increased length of day, such as from 7.30am to 9pm, to carry out the required procedures within a day, resulting in reduced savings in total labour costs, particularly if overtime payments are required.
4. Day cases may need separate dedicated recovery rooms, which in turn may require additional capital expenditure.
5. Capital savings from the reduction in overnight stays may only be achieved if the volume of transfers to day cases is large enough to close whole wards or transfer their functions to other specialties.
6. Day surgery may be inappropriate for the growing population of elderly patients.
7. Day cases may result in higher costs of transport for each day's patients to be home within the day, and impose greater external costs on the patients' relatives, particularly if they are in employment, as well as additional costs on GPs and other community services.
8. There is likely to be a limited and declining availability of informal carers to look after day-case patients after their discharge, in the face of prevailing social trends of a higher divorce rate and increasing numbers of single parents and single-person households.
9. Increasing the nominal number of day cases by opening patient hotels close to the hospital may simply shift the cost of recovery time to the patient without any reduction in total costs.

10. The provision of more day-case facilities is likely to result in an increased volume of patients treated rather than a reduction in total costs.
11. There may be greater risks to patients if there are complications after the operation when they have been discharged within the day, with any initial cost savings lost if readmission is necessary.

The above considerations will limit the extent to the NHS Executive's (1994) suggested target of 60 per cent of all elective surgery being carried out by day cases is both realistic and desirable. Similar considerations apply to the desirability of the increased use of laparoscopic or minimally invasive surgery (MIS), which a recent report (Cushieri 1994) for the Department of Health and Scottish Home and Health Department predicted would account for 70 per cent of all surgical operations within ten years (Bloor and Maynard 1994), and which some (e.g. Wickham 1994) have advocated as a main source of reductions in lengths of hospital stay. The net benefits of such a rapid expansion in the use of MIS are reduced by the following factors:

1. MIS requires expensive new capital equipment (Kesteloot and Penninckx 1993) to make use of fibre optics, micro-robotics and laser technology.
2. MIS is also likely to require the use of more highly skilled labour, such as consultants rather than junior doctors, and may require more time in the operating theatre (Cushieri 1993), in order to carry out the more delicate key-hole surgery and more sophisticated anaesthetics that MIS involves.
3. The use of the new laparoscopic procedures makes possible additional surgery that was not previously feasible, thereby potentially raising total costs (Banta 1993).
4. The increased use of MIS requires substantial changes to, and investment in, the training of surgeons, with less scope for the use of junior doctors training on the job in carrying out the new procedures (Wickham 1994).
5. MIS can involve greater risks if surgeons are insufficiently trained or operations do not go according to plan. A recent survey by the Royal College of Surgeons found that many surgeons were practising the new keyhole surgical techniques without sufficient training (*The Times*, 2 June 1994), with claims that 'at least six patients have died and many other have suffered serious post-operative complications following botched procedures' from the use of the new techniques (*Daily Telegraph*, 23 June 1994).
6. The cost of litigation resulting from the unsuccessful and inappropriate use of MIS can be substantial.
7. The use of MIS for many surgical operations has not been adequately evaluated as to its clinical and economic effectiveness (Banta 1993),

with the few randomized controlled trials that have been carried out confirming only some of the claimed benefits of MIS (Pearson 1994).

To some extent offsetting the above disadvantages may be an element of improved labour productivity from learning-by-doing, and falling average capital cost per case, as the volumes of day cases and MIS increase. In addition, a greater volume of day cases may in part succeed in relaxing the capital constraint on increased output from the availability of beds, thereby enabling the existing labour force to be used more intensively.

As Figure 6.3 demonstrates, the use of day cases was increasing substantially even before the NHS review. The future growth of day cases and MIS is itself largely in the hands of purchasers, i.e. district health authorities (DHAs) and the new area health commissions. A similar growth in reported activity generally in the Hospital and Community Health Services (HCHS) branch of the NHS, as reflected in the rise in its cost-weighted activity index (CWAI) in Figure 6.3, was evident well before the NHS review in 1989. Achieving further increases in day cases and MIS, even where these are desirable, is, however, dependent upon having available a sufficient quantity of skilled medical manpower, including consultant surgeons, anaesthetists and nurses, willing to work in the NHS for moderate wage rates, alongside sufficient funds for further capital investment where needed.

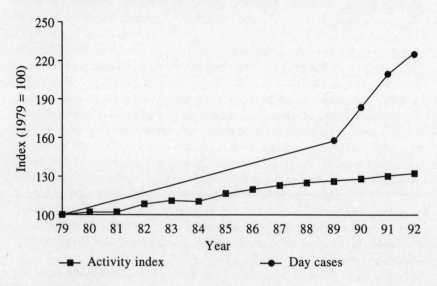

Source: DoH (1994).

Figure 6.3   The growth of day cases and the CWAI in the NHS

A further possible direction for improving the use of labour and capital in the NHS is through changes in the skill-mix of nursing and medical staff. One possibility is the substitution of lower-grade, and hence lower-cost, nursing staff for more highly qualified hospital nursing staff. However, the results of detailed studies by Carr-Hill et al. (1992) and Bagust et al. (1992) suggest that there are no substantial cost savings to be had from such skill-mix changes without threatening a reduction in the quality of patient care.

An additional possibility here is the substitution of practice nurses for more of the work of GPs, as advocated by Maynard and Walker (1993). The use of practice nurses has indeed trebled in the NHS since 1988. However, rather than providing a direct substitute for the existing labour of GPs, they have been used mainly to expand primary care services in the directions of meeting targets for child immunization and cervical cytology screening, minor surgery, and the provision of health promotion and other clinics, for which GPs receive additional payments under their revised, post-1990, contracts (Atkin and Hirst 1994). However, a recent study by Atkin and Hirst (1994) concluded that: 'It is not clear … whether, and to what extent, practice nurses' activities represent value for money', with Scott and Maynard (1991) criticizing many of these new services for being 'of dubious cost effectiveness'.

Another possible source of reduction in labour costs is through the greater use of competitive tendering in the NHS for services such as laundry and cleaning, so that internal labour has to compete with outside contractors for the contracts. However earlier cost improvement programmes, that were in operation before the NHS Review, have already introduced extensive competitive tendering, often with mixed results in terms of the quality of service that resulted. A King's Fund Institute (1989) study concluded that these programmes have been insufficiently monitored to conclude that the cost savings were achieved with no loss in quality of service. In addition, one would expect that the cost reductions which were easiest to achieve are those which were selected early on in the cost improvement programmes. The law of diminishing returns suggests that any further extensions of competitive tendering, such as to hospital laboratory services, are likely to be even more problematic in terms of substantial cost reductions being achievable without loss of quality of service.

The improved use of capital resources
A further possible source of improved efficiency in the NHS is through the greater utilization of specialized capital and labour resources, including operating theatres and staff. Earlier studies, such as NAO (1987), found that even within a standard 9–5 working day existing operating theatres were used only 50–60 per cent of the available time. However the limiting factor on their use was often the availability of key staff, such as anaesthetists, to avoid can-

celled sessions, together with sufficient revenue funding to hire staff for more planned sessions. Given sufficient additional funding to cover the additional marginal staffing costs involved, significantly greater throughput may then be possible in some cases. This is particularly so where improved scheduling and coordination of the use of beds, operating theatres, and specialized staff is achieved through improved bed and theatre management (see Audit Commission 1991b, 1992b).

The more intensive use of existing capital resources may also be achieved through improved estate management and space utilization. Scope for savings of some £300–500 million a year were indicated by one earlier NAO (1988) study, including energy savings from improved space utilization.

Further improvements in the management of existing capital assets may well be possible through the improved maintenance and replacement of existing assets. Largely as a reflection of past patterns of capital expenditure, and the subsequent neglect of maintenance and replacement needs (see Mayston 1990b), the NHS now faces a substantial maintenance time-bomb, with backlog maintenance expenditure requirements standing at an estimated £2.2 billion in England alone (*Guardian*, 8 November 1993).

As the experience of Wessex and West Midlands Regional Health Authorities shows, there is also a need for improved project management, in the investment of substantial amounts of new capital resources in projects such as new computer systems (see NAO 1990; PAC 1993). Similarly, the physical nature of many NHS hospital sites, as a mixture of sub-optimal size buildings resulting from penny-packet schemes approved whenever small amounts of capital were available, testifies to the need for greater efficiency in the management over time in new capital resources. A similar message emerges from cases such as Shropshire District Health Authority (Harvey-Jones 1990), where new hospitals have been acquired in addition to existing capital facilities without sufficient revenue resources to run both the new and existing hospitals at an efficient level.

The closures and disposals of hospitals, such as long-stay mental institutions, also provide scope in some cases for revenue and capital savings. However, as the Care in the Community programme illustrates, the quality of care may suffer as a result. The rundown in the number of long-stay beds in the NHS means that facilities are often now not available even for severe cases of schizophrenia, with several much publicized cases of resulting murder in the community. One estimate (Palmer 1994) is that one in seven of the 180,000 individuals nationally who suffer from schizophrenia commits suicide. This proportion is likely to be increased by a lack of adequate community psychiatric nurses and community facilities. In contrast, good-quality community care often requires significant new capital facilities and additional labour resources in the form of community nurses.

The capital savings from closing old long-stay sites are themselves only released when all patients are discharged from the site. This includes higher-dependency patients who in some cases should not be released into the community. While the cash generated by such asset sales has been substantial in some cases, such as at Banstead in prime stockbroker belt Surrey, this is far from true in all cases. The threat of compulsory purchase by the Home Office seeking to use several of the sites released as new prison sites, and falling land values after the collapse of the property boom of the 1980s, have both limited the capital receipts achieved. The fact that many regional capital building programmes in the NHS were in large part dependent on the income generated by such land sales points to both the overall shortage of new capital in the NHS and the dangers of finance-driven closures of existing long-stay institutions.

While technological change and increased medical knowledge frequently set up an increased demand for health care labour and capital, this need not always be the case. The discovery of the effectiveness of the humble aspirin in treating not only headaches but also heart disease and a wide range of other conditions can in contrast reduce the demand for more expensive drugs and treatments, and the associated need for specialized labour to administer them. The recent discovery that duodenal ulcers, gastric cancers and heart disease may have their origin in *helicobacter pylori* bacterial infection that can be treated relatively cheaply by antibiotics may reduce the demand for more labour-intensive surgical interventions or long courses of consultations and treatment (Mendall et al. 1994). Similarly the use of a simple chemical patch to reduce premature contractions can lessen the risk of premature births, with their resultant high demands on specialized labour and capital facilities. This measure can prove cost-effective in both reducing infant mortality and reducing the labour and capital costs incurred.

Will greater competition in the labour market help?
Our above discussion of the possibility of further reducing costs in the NHS suggests that there may be some limited scope for cost reductions, though this will require careful management and evaluation if the quality of care is not to suffer. Particularly where increases in efficiency are used to treat a greater volume of patients, the achievement of these efficiencies is, however, dependent upon the availability of sufficient skilled labour at a reasonable price. Will greater competition in the NHS labour market help to bring this about?

The city of York, where for many years there were only one or two large dominant employers of many types of labour, illustrates that greater competition in the labour market does not necessarily reduce labour costs. Instead greater competition can undermine the power of a single dominant purchaser of labour, i.e. a *monopsonist*, to reduce the price of labour below that which would prevail if competition for labour were to exist. The NHS as a whole is indeed at present a single dominant purchaser of several key types of health care labour, including 395,000 nurses and midwives, and 39,000 hospital doctors. With a total workforce of some 800,000, the NHS is one of the largest employers in the whole of Europe. As we have seen, labour costs are by far the largest component of total NHS costs. The NHS review itself was initiated in large part as a governmental response to the immediate funding pressures on the NHS that resulted from an annual round of wage settlements. Yet the only reference which the NHS review (DoH 1989a) made to the all-important labour market was its proposal to permit increased competition in the NHS labour market by allowing the new NHS self-governing trusts to 'be free to settle the pay and conditions of their staff, including doctors, nurses and others covered by national pay agreements' and thereby depart from these national pay agreements by greater local pay determination.

Acting on their own, as they are now able to do, NHS trusts have an incentive to hire labour up to the point where its marginal benefit equals the wage, putting greater upward pressure on labour demand and wages than under a monopsony where the marginal benefit of labour is equated to the marginal cost of labour. The latter differs significantly from the wage when, as in the NHS, a large quantity of labour is involved. Without rigidly enforced wage guidelines, decentralized NHS trusts have an incentive to undermine NHS monopsony power, just as the different members of a cartel have an incentive acting alone to destabilize the cartel, and thereby undermine the monopoly which would have remained stable had it remained under unified control.

The resultant higher wage under a decentralized competitive decision-making process compared to the monopsony wage may offset any cost reductions from the above efficiency gains. Even if the NHS faces some degree of monopoly power on the supply side of the NHS labour market (such as from the British Medical Association, the Royal College of Anaesthetists, or the Royal College of Nurses), monopsony power by the NHS in itself helps to provide countervailing power to reduce the resulting efficiency loss from monopoly. In contrast, abandoning NHS monopsony power by giving greater freedom to NHS trusts for local pay determination tends in itself to permit the monopoly power freer rein, although union power may itself to some extent be undermined by the greater fragmentation which local pay bargaining can involve. The importance of containing NHS labour costs is underlined by the fact that it would require a wage rise of only around 1.9 per cent to completely outweigh the annual new cost improvements that proved feasible before the NHS review (see Mayston 1990a).

Achieving the cost-reducing benefits of monopsony power then requires either central NHS control over wage determination by NHS trusts and other providers, and hence some form of collectivization of the supply side, or detailed central control over the prices which purchasers in the NHS are permitted to pay providers. Such price control would represent an attempt to achieve indirect monopsony power in the labour market through price control in the health care product market.

The above discussion implies that there may be distinct advantages to remaining with the public 'integrated' model discussed in Hurst (1996), particularly if managerial attention can be focused directly on the above sources of possible efficiency gains. Any move towards greater use of the 'public contract' model, such as has been involved in the NHS reforms, that widens the separation between public funding bodies and providing agencies risks reducing central monopsony power in the labour market, unless central price control is exercised over contract prices. To some extent offsetting the advantages of central monopsony power, however, may give greater scope for productivity bargaining from the wider use of local pay determination, although productivity agreements are still possible under centralized wage determination.

The extent to which greater competition in the labour market will cause wages to rise is greater under situations of excess demand in the labour market. In recent years both the recession and a shedding of nurses and other specialized staff in some parts of the NHS have limited labour market pressure. The result has been a significant fall in the turnover rate for nurses, with a consequent substantial saving in training and dislocation costs.

However, once the economy fully recovers from recession, and the retention rate of trained nurses falls to its former levels, these costs may rise significantly, particularly if trained nurses leave the NHS for private health care. A recent study by the Institute of Manpower Studies (Buchan and Seccombe 1991), for instance, found that a 10 per cent increase in its nurse turnover rate produced a cost increase of £210,000 per annum for a typical 350-bed hospital. With the added factor of greater competition between NHS trusts in the labour market, nurses, junior doctors and other medical staff will be able to cross town for a higher wage for a similar job, unless non-competitive wage guidelines are introduced to limit this process.

The scope for excess demand to develop in the UK health care labour market will also be increased by the proposed reduction in the previously excessive number of hours worked by many NHS junior hospital doctors, and by the recommendations of the Calman Report (1993) for less years of on-the-job training for junior doctors and more years of formal medical education to be given by senior doctors outside patient care. It will be further increased by any funded expansion in the volume and range of treatments offered in the NHS in response to an ageing population and technological change. The combination of these factors has been estimated by the British Orthopaedic Association (1995) to require at least a twofold increase in the number of consultant orthopaedic surgeons in the NHS. The planned further expansion of day cases, and of MIS, will similarly add further labour market pressure in key areas, such as in the demand for consultant surgeons and anaesthetists, where the available supply in the short run is relatively inelastic.

Labour market pressure on the NHS may also be increased by a number of other factors. The first is if the recent changes in the NHS produce greater stress, lower job satisfaction, less security and lower social motivation amongst its workforce, all of which can drive up the effective price that the NHS has to pay for its labour in the long term. One recent survey by the BBC2 *Public Eye* programme, for instance, found that some 40 per cent of GPs want to leave the NHS because of the increased stress they are experiencing as a result of the changes made by the NHS review. The suicides of two GPs were attributed by their widows at recent inquests to increased pressure of work following the NHS reforms (*The Times*, 16 June 1994).

A second factor is the influence of demographic trends due to the very large predicted drop in the ratio (from 1.43:1 in 1986 to 0.93:1 by 2025) between the number of 16–29-year-olds, from whom many nursing staff are drawn, and the number of over-65-year-olds (see Mayston 1990a). If the unemployment situation does ease in the economy at large for this age group, the combined effect of an increased difficulty of recruiting and retaining nurses and the greater demand for nursing from the ageing population may then cause development of excess demand for nurses. The likelihood of this is made even greater by the reductions that the Department of Health itself has made in recent years in the NHS intake of student nurses, which has fallen by 35 per cent between 1983 and 1993, and by a further 12 per cent during 1993–94 (Snell 1995).

A third factor is the introduction of greater financial incentives for NHS managers and clinicians to encourage patients into more expensive private health care as a result of the greater concern of NHS purchasers for improving their reported performance indicators, and the greater financial pressures on more autonomous NHS trusts in the new competitive NHS internal market.

One prime case where the NHS now has a strong financial incentive to divert patients into expensive private care is that of nursing care for the elderly. Particularly with the run-down in recent years of the capital stock of NHS long-stay beds, purchasers in the new NHS internal market have a strong financial incentive to seek to shift these relatively expensive patients off their NHS budgets and on to local authority social service budgets or on to private finance from accumulated lifetime personal savings. The NHS purchaser makes a substantial financial gain from such cost-shifting. In addition, NHS providers improve their reported performance indicators of throughput and finished consultant episodes (FCEs) through their resultant ability to substitute many day cases for one long-stay case.

This substitution will, moreover, significantly increase the *reported* level of hospital activity in the NHS in the published cost-weighted activity index (CWAI), largely as a result of the way in which the CWAI is constructed. A very high percentage (69.9 per cent) of the activity index is accounted for by the sub-component: 'All inpatient episodes and day cases' (see Mayston 1994). Within this vast sub-component, all episodes and cases are counted in units of FCEs, unweighted within this large sub-component by any consideration of cost or complexity. The policy of steadily discharging long-stay patients and using the expenditure released to expand the number of day cases then produces a much more dramatic increase in the *reported* activity index than if different forms of treatment had been weighted by their cost and complexity within this very large sub-component.

Even aside from the run-down of NHS long-stay care, increased competition and financial pressure on NHS managers, and the greater use of performance-related pay, may encourage a greater throughput of patients by volume and reduced length of stay, but with the quality of care possibly compromised. The imperfect nature of the performance indicators by which the output of NHS trusts and managers are judged is illustrated by the scope for manipulation which exists for increasing reported FCEs by passing patients more often between different departments and consultants within a hospital (see Seng et al. 1993).

While the greater use of clinical audits may help to ameliorate this problem, the imperfect nature of auditing is emphasized by the difficulties which have arisen in the generally simpler context of auditing private sector financial reports (see Mayston 1993). These difficulties are likely to increase with any increased divergence between the interests of managers or clinicians and the interests of those who they are appointed to serve, from the greater managerial pressure for improving reported performance indicators that now exists within the NHS.

Doubts among potential patients about the quality of care that is available in the NHS may lead over time to a higher level of demand for private health care. The problematic nature of the interface between individual NHS consultants and their own private work for private patients is emphasized by Yates (1995). It would appear possible to encourage a greater demand for private treatment by presenting NHS patients with longer waiting lists, and a declining availability of care, of reasonable quality and timeliness, within the NHS. What seems less widely appreciated is the scope that now exists for the new more autonomous NHS trusts to find a common interest with NHS consultants in the expansion of private health care within private pay beds in NHS trusts. This can both generate additional revenue for the individual NHS trust and enable each trust to offer individual consultants higher rates of direct remuneration and a greater volume of private patients, in return for limiting more strictly the consultants' own freelance private work. While such a policy is not explicitly part of the declared objective of NHS purchasers, the financial problems of NHS purchasers are also eased, at least in the short run, by the lower volume of demand from NHS patients that results from the greater substitution of private treatment.

In the long run, NHS trusts may well find private work significantly more profitable and less risky than reliance upon the uncertain future financial position and purchasing decisions of individual NHS purchasing authorities, with a consequent incentive to seek to expand further their private pay-bed activity. The effect of such an expansion in demand for private health care is likely to be to increase health care labour market pressure, with likely long-run increases in wage rates and costs for NHS purchasers. This effect will be even greater if there is any tendency for a higher level of 'supplier-induced demand' (Reinhardt 1985) under the financial incentives associated with private health care compared to those in the NHS.

The worst of all outcomes from the viewpoint of the NHS is then a downward spiral in which the quality and timeliness of care for NHS patients declines in the face of limited budgets, high staff turnover and rising wage rates, with patients increasingly turning to private health care to avoid declining quality of care in the NHS. This in turn is likely to drain more labour from the NHS, and cause wage rates and costs to rise further under increased competition for medical staff from private patients. Falling quality of care in the NHS may also further encourage nursing and medical staff to seek to transfer into private health care in order to maintain their own desired professional standards of care. The acceleration in recent years of the numbers of dentists in the UK wanting to switch out of the NHS and into private dental care (RBDDR 1994) emphasizes that the previously dominant position of the NHS in the health care labour market cannot be taken for granted, and can be undermined by an expanding demand for private health care in response to falling quality of care in the NHS. Once initiated, this process may be very difficult to reverse.

In terms of economic theory there are, then, serious questions raised about the *stability* of any more competitive health care labour market. The title of Henry Aaron's (1991) Brookings Institute study, *Serious and Unstable Condition*, of the cost escalation problems of the more competitive US health care system, underlines the fact that questions of stability and the risk of cost escalation in health care systems are not simply theoretical issues.

Maintaining the quality of care in the NHS then offers the best safeguard against such instability. A failure to fund the NHS sufficiently to maintain its quality of care can itself represent a form of economic inefficiency, through the government not respecting adequately the willingness of its citizens to pay for adequate health care. Such neglect can be at least as great a form of economic inefficiency as any other. The impact of such neglect on the welfare of patients, pressured into paying for higher-cost private health care out of accumulated private savings or into means-tested social security, and on the total costs of the UK health care and social security system, is likely to be detrimental.

As we have noted above, the rate of productivity growth in the NHS that is indicated by the use of the CWAI as the overall index of HCHS activity in the Department of Health's own Annual Report (DoH 1994) tends to overstate the true underlying rate of productivity growth. A lower achievable rate of productivity growth in the NHS implies the need for a greater rate of increase of the level of funding of the NHS, if the quality of care is to be maintained, to keep pace with increases in real wages and the associated relative price effect. This becomes even more strongly so if the main form of productivity growth in the NHS in recent years, that of day cases, is problematic in its future potential.

Competitive markets for capital?
In approaching the issue of whether markets for capital in the NHS are desirable, we may first note that competitive markets can in general only be shown to be efficient through the standard theorems of welfare economics (see e.g. Gravelle and Rees 1992) if these markets are *complete*. In our present context, this means that *futures markets* have to exist for the delivery of health care by supply-side providers. In practical terms, this means that purchasers must be willing to offer providers long-term contracts for their future output. However, the contracts on offer under the new internal market arrangements of the NHS are typically only for a year or so, far less than the life of many NHS capital assets. When adequate futures markets do not exist, we know that major inefficiencies can result from uncoordinated investment decisions that fail to achieve their expected benefits. Simple textbook cobweb models of market behaviour illustrate both the likelihood of uncoordinated decentralized investment decisions failing to achieve their expected benefits in the absence of futures markets, and the risk of market instability over time.

The supply lags and lack of forward markets that in part generate such instability and inefficiencies also characterize health care markets for human capital. The training of additional manpower takes several years and involves a high investment cost. Individual prospective nurses and doctors, and the NHS, must all make major decisions regarding expensive investments in human capital. Again one cannot necessarily rely upon market forces alone to bring about efficiency. Rather there is a need for some degree of coordination between training places offered and anticipated future demand, though with scope for improvements in precisely how this anticipated future demand is estimated, as in Maynard and Walker (1993).

Similarly one cannot expect efficiency to result from a system where, as at present, the NHS trains doctors and nurses free of charge for the private sector which then employs without recompense to the NHS. The *public good* aspects of training, whereby other hospitals can poach labour trained by one hospital without necessarily contributing to these training costs, also imply that the training of nurses and doctors cannot simply be left to competitive markets. Rather adequate specific funding is needed for the training of nurses and doctors, and for associated medical schools and teaching hospitals, if these institutions are not to suffer in the internal market from their associated higher costs, not only direct training costs, but also supportive research, which individual purchasers of health care may be unwilling to pay for directly.

Where hospitals are able to differentiate their product by location, unrestricted free-market entry can also result in *excess capacity*, as under standard monopolistic competition models in economic theory. The problem of inefficient excess capacity has arisen both in the private health care sector in the UK and in the market-oriented US health care system, where it was found desirable to require Certificates of Need before granting permission for new hospitals to avoid further excess capacity.

Capital investment in health care facilities tends also to be associated with the existence of indivisibilities and fixed costs. These in turn generate *economies of scale* under which the marginal cost of further operations and health care treatments is less than the average cost. Efficiency typically requires prices to be set at marginal cost. When marginal cost is less than average cost, this can be shown to result in a financial loss for the hospital, even though it is setting efficient prices and may be operating at the lowest cost possible for its volume of output. A market system of competing suppliers, in the presence of economies of scale, is also then unstable, tending to lead to local monopoly on the supply side. Prices will as a result be set at monopolistic levels above their most efficient level, with the supply of health care at less than its optimal level.

The cost advantages of local monopolies may be further increased by the investment required to introduce technological change, as in the expansion of day cases and laparoscopic (key-hole) surgery. Cushieri (1993), for example, estimates that the total throughput of laparoscopic cholecystectomies required before it becomes financially beneficial to invest in the new capital equipment required for laparoscopic, rather than open, surgery, is 140 patients a year. The need for more skilled labour, such as consultant surgeons and anaesthetists, to carry out the new techniques in association with the new capital equipment further weakens the ability of smaller district general hospitals (DGHs) to offer effective competition against larger local monopolies as potential providers of many surgical procedures.

The tendency towards economies of scale in the NHS may be increased by considerations of learning-by-doing and quality variations, as well as indivisibilities. The skill and experience of individual surgeons, and resultant quality of care and lack of clinical complications for individual patients, is likely to be positively related to the volume of operations they perform in a given category. Surgical death rates were found by Kind (1990) to be significantly negatively related to the degree of specialization on surgical work within each hospital. The existence of excess capacity in many existing NHS hospitals, as reported in NAO (1987), further confirms the potential for reaping economies of scale and falling average costs from concentrating activity in a limited number of existing hospitals, rather than from their competitive duplication.

A concept related to economies of scale is that of economies of scope. This means that it is cheaper to produce several things together under one single producer rather than to produce them separately by different producers. Since hospitals are multi-product producers, supplying many different forms of treatment, economies of scope may well arise on the supply side of health care, particularly where different forms of treatment share the same capital facilities and specialized labour. A natural monopoly is then one where a monopoly is the lowest-cost producer of a given set of outputs, able to secure both economies of scale and economies of scope compared to many small competing producers. Except where the population density is particularly high, many existing district general hospitals are *de facto* local monopolies for many forms of treatment, once considerations of ease of access are taken into account. To determine whether or not they are lowest-cost natural monopolies would require a detailed examination of the extent of economies of scale and scope involved.

The question then arises as to how far one can short-circuit this detailed examination by subjecting such local monopolies to competition, or more generally, potential competition, in the hope that efficiency will be thereby generated. If the local health care market were to be made *contestable*, there would be freedom for any potential supplier to invest in new additional capital facilities to supply the market, if it appears profitable to do so. Such a philosophy has underlain the deregulation of US airlines and similar activities where capital is 'on wheels', and an airline may costlessly move its capital assets, in the form of aircraft, to new routes if it appears profitable to do so, with the threat of such potential entry placing downward pressure on the prices an incumbent producer can charge.

However, in the presence of economies of scale and scope, and of sunk capital costs in existing hospitals, there is no guarantee in general that even a perfectly efficient natural monopoly will be able to remain financially viable and avoid bankruptcy in the face of such contestability. An example of an economy of scope in the NHS arises if it is cheaper to run an accident and emergency unit alongside acute wards, so that specialists are readily on hand to treat emergency cases. The acute wards themselves may experience economies of scope by treating both complicated cases and more routine cases together, thereby making more intensive use of the specialized capital and labour resources of the acute wards and operating theatres than if they were to treat only the complicated cases. The district general hospital, if of sufficient size, may well then be a natural local monopoly able to secure these economies of scope and to supply the local health care needs, without excessive transport costs for patients, in the least-cost way.

One way to open up this natural monopoly to contestability is to allow GP fundholders, under their new freedom, to make their own purchasing decisions, to offer contracts to new clinics set up to carry out only the routine treatments. However, in doing so, they may then bankrupt the district general hospital. While the new clinics may be able to secure partial economies of scale in the routine operations, they will do so by undermining the economies of scope of the DGH, when they take away its former volume of routine operations. By such 'cherry-picking' they inflict a *cost externality* on the DGH in a way which is not taken into account by the new contracting arrangements, once there is decentralized decision-making by different GP fundholders. There may then be no 'sustainable prices' that enable the natural monopoly of the district general hospital to survive financially, by being able to quote prices which deter new entrants from such cherry-picking while still avoiding financial losses.

Since there is no guarantee here that even efficient hospitals will be financially viable, one cannot assume that competition and freedom of capital investment into a 'contestable' health care market will result in only inefficient hospitals being made bankrupt. The inclusion of capital into the production process inherently involves *intertemporal* considerations. That there may well be no sustainable prices to ensure that even efficient natural monopolies survive in a contestable market system is stressed by Baumol, Panzar and Willig (1982, pp. 405–6):

> Some observers have ... been led to conjecture that unsustainability is a pathological phenomenon which has more interest as an analytical curiosum than as a phenomenon in the world of reality. ... We find that all this changes drastically in an intertemporal setting. Unsustainability can come closer to being the rule rather than the exception. ... In the intertemporal case, ... we find that the domain of the invisible hand can be far more limited than intuition may have led us to suspect.

Often there may well be no sustainable solutions and the market mechanism may well produce an intertemporal allocation of resources that is patently inefficient.

Once there is no sustainable set of contract prices that will protect even an efficient hospital from financial insolvency, the two main problems produced are first the 'vulnerability of [the] industry to forms of entry that raise total production costs' and '"disorderly" evolution ... that is, a time path of evolution of industry structure and utilization of capital that can be said to be inconsistent with intertemporal efficiency in resource allocation' (ibid., pp. 348–9).

A more competitive market in capital to supply the NHS can also produce problems of increased costs in a number of other directions. The first of these is the increased *transactions costs* which a system of contracts between numerous different suppliers and purchasers generates. Keeping track of the post-code of each patient's address for the purpose of billing, or for monitoring the fulfilment of contacts with different purchasing DHAs, can then be as important financially for a hospital as treating the patient.

Payment systems can themselves create incentives for cost escalation. This is particularly so if they are retrospectively based on the amount of treatment actually carried out. On the other hand, prospective payment systems that offer a fixed advanced payment for different categories of treatment can risk compromising quality of care as providers seek to make a profit or accumulate financial surpluses by cutting back on costs within the fixed payment. In addition, there can arise the danger of cost escalation through 'Diagnostically Related Group (DRG)-creep' due to the resulting financial incentive to classify patients in higher fee categories than they would otherwise be placed in. Some US studies (e.g. Kahn et al. 1990) suggest that these dangers need not be great, although avoiding them may itself involve substantial monitoring and auditing costs.

The substantial additional capital expenditure on new computer systems and additional labour costs of information technology specialists that have accompanied the introduction of the internal market have also produced a greater *dependency* of the NHS on the proper operation of these new computer systems. Doubts about the cost-effectiveness of the capital investment in such new computer systems are raised in a number of reports. A study by Packwood et al. (1991) failed to find any significant benefits from the substantial investment in computers and manpower that was involved in the resource management initiative (RMI). The RMI, and the associated large-scale capital investment in new computer systems, was nonetheless subsequently extended across the whole country by the NHS reforms despite these negative findings. The Comptroller and Auditor General (NAO 1992) found that the regional information systems plan computer project of Wessex

Regional Health Authority, which cost in total up to £63 million, was subsequently abandoned 'without any significant benefit having accrued to the region'. The National Audit Office (1990) has also reported more widely on the difficulties of introducing an internal market into the NHS when this involves reliance upon the proper operation of new computer systems.

Managed competition?

The above problems involving capital under a more competitive market should not obscure the fact that there were many problems with the management of NHS capital before the NHS review. Partly these stemmed from the limited total availability of capital to the NHS under constrained overall levels of public expenditure. Introducing more private capital into the supply of health care to the NHS then relaxes this constraint to some extent. However it also poses the question of whether that capital could not be raised more cheaply through government borrowing, with greater value for money thereby achieved. If the total level of the government's public sector borrowing requirement (PSBR) is constrained at a given total level for macroeconomic reasons, such as the control of inflation, increasing capital expenditure on the NHS by private finance is essentially a back-door method of relaxing this constraint, at a potentially more expensive price than directly through the PSBR.

Previous problems with the use of NHS capital involved not only the total availability of capital to the NHS but also inefficiencies in the management of the given total amount of capital resources (including both new investment and existing assets) that were available to the NHS. These difficulties are discussed at length in Mayston (1990b). One of the main sources of these difficulties is the conflict between efficient intertemporal capital resource utilization and the existing control mechanisms for public expenditure on the NHS, namely those of annual cash budgeting, annual cash limits and annual cash-flow accounting. Unfortunately, the system of capital charging that was introduced by the NHS review, as part of an attempt to manage the internal market by imposed rules, does nothing to overcome this basic problem, but instead creates additional new problems which we discuss below.

The main problems in the management of NHS capital resources before the NHS Review were:

1. An imbalance between revenue and capital expenditure at the local level, so that new capital assets were acquired without sufficient revenue to operate them efficiently.
2. The under-utilization of existing assets.
3. Accumulating back-log maintenance and replacement expenditure requirements for the existing capital stock.

The system of capital charging introduced by the NHS review has two main parts. The first is a straight-line depreciation charge. The second is an interest charge at 6 per cent above inflation. Both are calculated on the basis of 'the value' of the provider's capital assets, principally its land, and the hospital and equipment, where the latter two sets of assets are valued at their depreciated replacement cost (DRC).

The system operates differently for directly managed units (DMUs) and for NHS trusts. For DMUs, the resultant charge is paid in cash terms to the regional health authority. The district health authority which operates the DMU then receives back a 'capital-funding' cash payment, which may or may not offset the capital charge. Since the NHS review, the system has been in 'neutral' mode with the 'capital-funding' element set equal to the capital charge, so that it has no direct net effect.

NHS trusts, on the other hand, are not required to make any cash payments for their capital charge. Instead the charge enters into their accounts as an increased accounting cost through the depreciation and interest elements of the capital charge.

When the DMU capital-charging system is in 'neutral' mode, the main impact of the system is not to address the original main problems listed above. Instead its main impact is on:

4. The level of prices set by the provider in the internal market through the requirement in DoH (1989b) that the prices set by each provider should cover their average costs, inclusive of their capital charges.

With the advent of the Tomlinson Report on the future of London hospitals, and similar closure proposals elsewhere in the NHS, a knock-on effect of the main impact of the capital charging system on contract prices in the new internal market is then on:

5. Closure decisions for NHS hospitals and wards.

Table 3 of the Tomlinson (1992) Report, for instance, sought to identify 'the vulnerability of Inner London hospitals' to price competition in the internal market, when these prices are based upon 'Hospitals' actual costs, including capital charges' (ibid., p. 28). However capital charges are not 'an actual cost' but rather an accounting concoction introduced into the NHS by the NHS review.

The basis on which the capital charge for buildings is typically calculated, that of depreciated replacement cost, dates back to the system of current cost accounting that was itself rejected by much of the accountancy profession during the 1980s. The traditional purpose of capital accounting, on which the system of capital charging introduced into the NHS is based, has to do with a rather different objective to those of price setting and closure decisions. This is that of:

6.   Monitoring the stewardship of, and value for money obtained from, the capital assets held by the organization.

The issues involved in the points listed above all pose different questions for which different answers are appropriate (see Mayston 1992b). The main defect of the system of capital charging introduced by the NHS review is that it puts numbers which are appropriate to issue 6 in as incorrect answers to 4 and 5, without directly addressing the original problems 1, 2 and 3 at all. In doing so, it both wires up the electric plug incorrectly and leaves trailing loose wires.

That the numbers produced by the new NHS capital charging system are not the right ones to answer the pricing issue follows from our earlier discussion on the desirability of marginal cost pricing rather than average cost pricing. The inclusion of capital charges into prices with the requirement that is implicit in the Department of Health's (1989b) requirement that the hospital break even at these prices leads to *average cost pricing* rather than *marginal cost pricing*.

That the numbers produced by the new NHS capital charging system are not the right ones to answer the closure issue follows from an examination of the difference between depreciated replacement cost, which forms the basis of the asset valuation for the NHS capital-charging system for hospital buildings, and the more general notion of the *value to the business* that underlies current cost accounting valuations. We may show that the appropriate valuation basis for capital assets under the value to the business approach is only equal to depreciated replacement cost *if it is has already been decided not to dispose of the asset*. There is then an inherent logical contradiction in using capital charges based on depreciated replacement cost (DRC) *as the basis for decisions on closures*, in the way the Tomlinson Report would have us do, since the use of DRC already assumes *that closure will not take place*.

The valuation basis that is appropriate to the closure issue is not DRC but the net realizable value (NRV) of the asset. For many NHS assets, that have high costs of construction but few alternative uses, their net realizable value is significantly less than their depreciated replacement costs, reflecting a large element of *sunk costs* involved. Basing closure decisions incorrectly on DRC, in the way Tomlinson and the new NHS capital-charging system would have us do for hospital buildings, then leads to an excessive and inefficient number of hospital and ward closures compared to what use of the correct NRV method would entail.

A further problem with the new NHS capital-charging system, which we have argued is not correctly wired up, occurs if the power is later turned fully on, by making the system non-neutral. Such a step is indeed proposed under the new capital-charging system at some date in the not too distant future. Directly managed units will then have to find in cash out of their revenue income (that forms the life-blood of hospital financing) the difference between their capital charge and their capitation-weighted share of the total regional fund of capital charges received. Since the capital charge is levied as a mortgage at 6 per cent above inflation on the depreciated replacement cost of the hospital, the sums involved are not trivial. A 20-year-old hospital with a total expected useful life of 60 years and a replacement cost as new of £90 million, for instance, generates a capital charge per annum of £5.1 million per annum. This large sum must be found out of the hospital's revenue income (that would otherwise be spent on patient care) and its capital-funding element.

For any health authority having more capital stock than its population-weighted average for the region, the result is likely to be a substantial net cash charge, were its hospitals to remain directly managed. One health authority that might well have more capital stock than the population-weighted average is Shropshire, which acquired a new DGH at Telford before the NHS review, in addition to an older hospital in Shrewsbury. As John Harvey-Jones (1990) discovered on his visit there, even before the NHS review Shropshire DHA was experiencing significant revenue pressures in attempting to maintain a high level of utilization of its capital stock. A large capital charge in excess of the capital-funding inflow would make these revenue pressures even worse.

The interaction of the high capital charges with the break-even requirement to price at average cost would tend to push such hospitals into an unstable downward spiral. The higher prices set in an attempt to cover higher average costs will discourage purchaser demand, with the average costs rising even further as utilization of the fixed capital facilities then falls and the break-even level of prices rises even further. The result will be increasing excess capacity, cumulative cash-flow problems and a risk of insolvency. Again the fact that the capital charges for buildings are based on depreciated replacement cost valuations, rather than typically much lower net realizable value assessments, means that there is no guarantee that the outcome of such a process will be in line with economic efficiency.

Since the cash charge only applies to directly managed units, the claim made by the NHS review White Paper (DoH 1989a) that a level playing-field would be established between directly managed units and NHS trusts would also not be valid. Since, however, trusts are able to retain their cash surpluses (subject to any demands from HM Treasury for public dividend capital to be

paid out of this surplus), there may be a temptation for those trusts that start
ahead in this unstable process to invest in new capacity out of these cash
surpluses. The result may then be expensive new building being undertaken
at the same time as substantial excess capacity exists in sunk capital facilities
in other local hospitals, with low opportunity cost of using these existing
facilities.

Once the capital-charging system is made non-neutral, there is in addition
a strange externality in the system. In order to stay in line with the population-weighted average level of capital stock, all other hospitals in the region
have to close wards or make disposals if any one of them does. This will
encourage a further downward spiral of capital decline with no necessary
economic justification. Even in neutral mode, a similar strange externality
effect will operate through the interaction between capital charging and contract prices in the new internal market, under the Department of Health's
break-even constraint for both directly managed units and NHS trusts (DoH
1989b).

The situation is particularly acute in the case of large cities, such as
London, where land values tend to make capital charges for inner-city hospitals greater than those for hospitals further from the centre. The result of the
capital-charging system is then to threaten the financial solvency of inner-city
hospitals, either directly through the above cash-flow effects when the system
is in non-neutral mode, or indirectly through contract prices when the system
is in neutral mode, as at present.

In view of the above difficulties, there is an urgent need for a thorough
review of the operation and design of the system of capital charging that was
introduced under the NHS reforms. These difficulties are themselves made
worse by the interaction that currently exists between capital charges, pricing
decisions, cash-flows and financial solvency, with a defect in one having
knock-on effects on the others.

The relationship between capital charges and prices is made even more
complex once issues of cost allocation arise when different purchasers and
treatments make use of the same capital facilities. There is then no unique
answer to the accountant's overly simple question of what is 'the cost' of a
given form of treatment, with the correct answer depending on which of the
questions one is attempting to answer. Making the wrong connections between answers and questions, as the new NHS capital-charging system does,
again produces potentially dangerous results.

Evolutionary progress

We have noted above that the efficient operation of competitive markets
depends upon a number of assumptions, such as completeness of markets and
stability, that may well not hold in practice in health care. As we have seen,

there is then scope for cost escalation in associated labour and capital costs for health care when these assumptions do not hold. To avoid counterproductive changes, we need to return to base by recognizing that, despite a number of defects, the pre-review NHS nevertheless had the following major advantages which we risk losing at our peril:

1. Cost containment, through the imposition of cash limits on total NHS spending on hospital care.
2. Control over the solvency of individual hospitals, all of which were under the direct financial control of their district health authorities.
3. Monopsony power in the labour market.
4. Relatively low administrative and managerial costs.
5. A workforce with some degree of social motivation.

As we have noted above, there were, however, significant problems in the management of capital resources in the pre-review NHS. The question then arises as to whether one cannot make more evolutionary, incremental improvements in the management of NHS capital resources that avoid the above dangers of cost escalation from a wholescale move to a free-market system in capital and labour. As noted above, one of the main problems in the management of NHS capital resources is the conflict between efficient intertemporal capital resource utilization and the traditional control mechanisms for public expenditure on the NHS, that of annual cash budgeting, annual cash limits and annual cash-flow accounting. As advocated in Mayston (1990b and c), there is a system, based on the concept of *capital credits*, that addresses this underlying source of the difficulties directly, and permits the intertemporal optimization of capital and revenue resource utilization by individual health authorities.

The capital credit system involves the centre, through regional health authorities (or their successors, the new regional offices of the NHS Executive), acting as the banker for capital credit accounts for individual district health authorities (or their successors, the area health commissions). Each DHA receives an annual addition of credit income to its capital credit balance, made through a resource allocation formula that takes into account both the size and nature of its local population in determining its target capital stock and its existing endowment of capital stock. In this way the DHA's entitlement to new capital credits to make good over time any deficit between its target capital stock and its existing capital stock can be determined.

While a larger existing capital stock reduces its entitlement to additional new capital credits, this does not produce a cash charge for its existing capital stock which affects its contract prices or its financial solvency. It therefore overcomes the disadvantages of the existing NHS system of capital charges.

It also provides a medium within which individual purchasers and providers can accumulate surpluses or incur debt, while remaining within overall national cash limits for public expenditure control purposes. Moreover, it is consistent with a regional overview of where new capital facilities are desirable, and with regulation of where they are permitted. The regional banker is able to sanction, or otherwise, the authorization of capital expenditure in cash terms on any particular new project within overall regional cash limits. The capital credit system is consistent with any desired degree of *virement* between revenue income and capital credits. It can also readily monitor value for money for both purchasers and providers through capital accounting on the basis of lessor and lessee accounting respectively, as required by objective 6 above.

Given that excess capacity of capital facilities has been one of the main problems in NHS capital resource management, another incremental means of introducing some of the advantages of a market mechanism without many of its disadvantages is through an on-line 'Exchange and Mart' Prestel-type computer system for GPs and health authorities to tap into, in order to identify where there is current spare capacity for different types of operation (see Mayston 1992a). So long as the price quoted by a hospital with spare capacity covers marginal cost, in the way the hospital itself has an incentive to ensure without an elaborate accounting system or capital charging system, there will be scope for mutually beneficial gains between purchasers and providers from such short-term trading. Longer-term issues of which hospitals are to remain open can then be determined through the mechanisms of regulation and service planning. If there is evidence of inefficient management of a particular hospital, which as we have noted above is not the same thing as its financial solvency, then this is a case for replacing the existing management, rather than for closing down the hospital.

Two of the traditional advantages of open markets, and of 'Exchange and Mart' arrangements, are the low-cost basis of their operation and their ability to respond readily to short-term fluctuations in supply and demand. These advantages contrast with the managerially costly new internal market system in the NHS that is based upon yearly contracts that neither adequately meet the need for long-term forward markets nor provide short-term purchasing flexibility to make use of excess capacity. Instead the limited funds now available to purchasers for extra-contractual referrals (ECRs) significantly restrict their short-term flexibility. As we have seen, the imposition of average cost pricing and the lack of effective forward markets both limit considerably the efficiency gains from the introduction of the existing NHS internal market.

Conclusions

As we have seen, two major features of the NHS are that it is *labour-intensive* and *relatively low-cost* in terms of international comparisons. There may be some limited scope for further reductions in NHS costs in delivering the existing package of health care demands without compromising quality of care. However, there are also dangers of substantial upward pressures on both labour and capital costs from the introduction of changes in the operation of the NHS, including that of greater competition.

Science generally has moved beyond a simple deterministic view of the world in which small changes in one parameter necessarily produce small smooth changes in the other variables that characterize the state of the system. However, this rather simplistic view still characterizes much of the current dominant tradition of economics, that of neoclassical economics. Its primary tool of analysis is typically the Newtonian device of differential calculus, in which small changes in one parameter are typically assumed to be associated with small changes in other variables. In contrast, more recent developments in both chaos theory and catastrophe theory emphasize that even small perturbations to a system can dramatically change the behaviour of the system for the worse, in ways which may be very difficult to reverse once initiated. The NHS reforms represent major perturbations to the health care system of a nation, without scope for adequate debate or pilot experiments before many of the changes were made. As we have emphasized above, one cannot assume that the outcomes from such perturbations will either be stable or improve welfare.

One particular area which we have highlighted in this paper as in urgent need of review is that of the design and operation of the system of capital charging introduced by the NHS review. We have also urged caution in making the NHS labour market more competitive, with again the risk of counterproductive cost escalation and a downward spiral in the quality of care offered by the NHS. Competition in the supply of capital facilities can also result in instabilities and excessive levels of costs. While there are ways in which positive progress can be made, they need to be approached carefully and with adequate attention to detail. As with surgical interventions, simply rearranging the internal workings of a body without sufficient care, thought, and understanding of relevant branches of knowledge may prove counterproductive, particularly when that body is the health care system of a whole country.

References

Aaron, H.J. (1991), *Serious and Unstable Condition: Financing America's Health Care*, Washington, DC: Brookings Institute.

Atkin, K. and Hirst, M. (1994), 'Costing Practice Nurses: Implications for Primary Care', University of York, Centre for Health Economics, Discussion Paper 117.

Audit Commission (1990), *A Short Cut to Better Services: Day Surgery in England and Wales*, London: HMSO.

Audit Commission (1991a), *NHS Estate Management and Property Maintenance*, London: HMSO.

Audit Commission (199lb), *The Virtue of Patients: Making Best Use of Ward Nursing Resources*, London: HMSO.

Audit Commission (1992a), *All in a Day's Work*, London: HMSO.

Audit Commission (1992b), *Lying in Wait: The Use of Medical Beds in Acute Hospitals*, London: HMSO.

Bagust, A., Slack, R. and Oakley, J. (1992), *Ward Nursing Quality and Grade-Mix*, York: York Health Economics Consortium, University of York.

Banta, H.D. (1993), 'Minimally Invasive Surgery: Implications for Hospitals, Health Workers and Patients', *British Medical Journal*, **307**, 1546–9.

Baumol, W., Panzar, J. and Willig, R. (1982), *Contestable Markets and the Theory of Industry Structure*, New York: Harcourt Brace Jovanovich.

Bloor, K. and Maynard, A. (1992), *Rewarding Excellence? Consultants' Distinction Awards and the Need for Reform*, University of York, Centre for Health Economics, Discussion Paper 100.

Bloor, K. and Maynard, A. (1994), 'Through The Keyhole', *Health Service Journal*, 17 November, pp. 24–6.

British Orthopaedic Association (1995), *Consultant Staffing Requirements for an Orthopaedic Service in the National Health Service*, London: BOA.

Bryan, J. (1995), 'Daylight Savings', *Health Service Journal*, 16 February, pp. 3–4.

Buchan, J. and Seccombe, I. (1991), *Nurse Turnover Costs*, Report no. 212, Brighton: Institute of Manpower Studies.

Calman, K. (Chair) (1993), *Hospital Doctors: Training for the Future*, Report of the Working Group on Specialist Medical Training, London: Department of Health.

Carr-Hill, R., Dixon, P., Gibbs, I., Griffiths, M., Higgins, M., McCaughan D. and Wright K. (1992), 'Skill-Mix and the Effectiveness of Nursing Care', University of York, Centre for Health Economics, Occasional Paper.

Cushieri, A. (1993), 'Cost-Effectiveness of Endoscopic Surgery', *Health Economics*, **2**(4), 295–376.

Cushieri, A. (1994), *Minimal Access Surgery: Implications for the NHS*, Edinburgh: HMSO.

Department of Health (1989a), *Working For Patients*, Cm. 555, London: HMSO.

Department of Health (1989b), *Self-governing Hospitals: An Initial Guide*, London: HMSO.

Department of Health (1993), *Health and Personal Social Services Statistics for England*, (1993 edn), London: HMSO.

Department of Health (1994), *Departmental Report: The Government's Expenditure Plans 1994–95 to 1996–97*, London: HMSO.

Gravelle, H. and Rees, R. (1992), *Microeconomics* (2nd edn), Harlow: Longman.

Harvey-Jones, J. (1990), *Trouble Shooter*, London: BBC.

Hurst, J. (1996), 'The UK Health Service Reforms in An International Context', Chapter 2 of this volume.

Iliffe, S. and Munro, J. (1993), 'General Practitioners and Incentives', *British Medical Journal*, **307**, 1156–7.

Kahn, K.L., Rogers, W.H. and Rubenstein, L.V. (1990), 'Measuring Quality of Care With Explicit Process Criteria Before and After Implementation of the DRG-Based Prospective Payment System', *Journal of the American Medical Association*, **264**, 1969–73.

Kesteloot, D. and Penninckx, F. (1993), 'The Costs and Effects of Open Versus Laparoscopic Cholecystectomies', *Health Economics*, **2**(4), 295–376.

Kind, P. (1990), 'Outcome Measurement Using Hospital Activity Data: Deaths After Surgical Procedures', *British Journal of Survey*, **77**, 1399–402.

King's Fund Institute (1989), 'Efficiency in the NHS: A Study of Cost Improvement Programmes', King's Fund Institute, London, Occasional Paper No. 2.

Maynard, A. and Walker, A. (1993), 'Planning the Medical Workforce – Struggling Out of the Time Warp', University of York, Centre for Health Economics, Discussion Paper 105.

Mayston, D.J. (1990a), 'NHS Resourcing: A Financial and Economic Analysis', Chapter 3 in Culyer, A., Maynard, A. and Posnett, J. (eds), *Competition in Health Care*, London: Macmillan.

Mayston, D.J. (1990b), 'Managing Capital Resources in the NHS', Chapter 5 in Culyer, A., Maynard, A. and Posnett, J. (eds), *Competition in Health Care*, London: Macmillan, pp. 138–77.

Mayston, D.J. (1990c), 'Capital Charging and the Management of NHS Capital', NHS White Paper Occasional Paper, University of York, Centre for Health Economics, Occasional Paper 7.

Mayston, D.J. (1992a), 'Internal Markets, Capital and the Economics of Information', *Public Money and Management*, **12**, London: Public Finance Foundation, pp. 47–54.

Mayston, D.J. (1992b), 'Capital Accounting, User Needs and the Foundations of a Conceptual Framework for Public Sector Financial Reporting', *Financial Accountability and Management*, **8**, Oxford: Basil Blackwell, pp. 227–48.

Mayston, D.J. (1993), 'Principals, Agents and the Economics of Accountability in the New Public Sector', *Accounting, Accountability and Auditing Journal*, **6**(3), 68–96.

Mayston, D.J. (1994), *Output Indicators in the Public Services*, London: HM Treasury.

Mendall, M.A., Goggin, P., Molineaux, N., Levy, J., Toosy, T., Strachan, D., Camm, A. and Northfield, T. (1994), Relation of *Helicobacter Pylori* Infection and Coronary Heart Disease', *British Heart Journal*, **71**, 437–9.

National Audit Office (1987), *Use of Operating Theatres in the National Health Service*, HC 143, London: HMSO.

National Audit Office (1988), *Estate Management in the National Health Service*, HC 405, London: HMSO.

National Audit Office (1990), *Managing Computer Projects in the National Health Service*, HC 22, London: HMSO.

National Audit Office (1992), *Report of Comptroller and Auditor General on Department of Health Appropriation Accounts*, London: HMSO.

NHS Executive (1994), *Day Surgery Task Force Report and Toolkit Upgrade*, Leeds: NHS Executive.

Organization for Economic Cooperation and Development (1993), *OECD Health Systems*, I and II, Paris: OECD.

Packwood, T., Keen, J. and Buxton, M. (1991), *Hospitals in Transition*, Milton Keynes: Open University Press.

Palmer, A. (1994), 'Carnage in the Community', *The Spectator*, 7 May, pp. 9–11.

Pearson, V. (1994), *Minimal Access Surgery: A Review*, Bristol: Health Care Evaluation Unit, University of Bristol.

Public Accounts Committee (1993), *Wessex Regional Health Authority: Management of the Regional Information Systems Plan*, Minutes of Evidence, HC 658i, London: HMSO.

Reinhardt, U. (1985), 'The Theory of Physician-Induced Demand', *Journal of Health Economics*, **4**, 187–93.

Review Body on Doctors' and Dentists' Remuneration (1994), *Report*, Cm 2460, London: HMSO.

Scott, T. and Maynard, A. (1991), 'Will the New GP Contract Lead to Cost Effective Medical Practice?', University of York, Centre for Health Economics, Discussion Paper 82.

Seng, C., Lessof, L. and McKee, M. (1993), 'Who's on the Fiddle?', *Health Service Journal*, 7 January, 16–17.

Snell, J. (1995), 'Rules of Attraction', *Nursing Times*, **91**(8), 19.

Tomlinson, Sir B. (1992), *Report of the Inquiry Into London's Health Service Medical Education and Research*, London: HMSO.

Wickham, J.E.A. (1994), 'Minimally Invasive Surgery: Future Developments', *British Medical Journal*, **308**, 193–6.

Yates, J. (1995), *Serving Two Masters: Consultants the NHS and Private Medicine*, London: Channel Four Television.

7 Is there adequate funding of health care?

Alistair McGuire

Introduction

Not so long ago it seemed a widely held belief that the National Health Service (NHS) was one of, if not the best health care service in the world. More recently it has been increasingly subject to criticism. While the delivery of service is still considered to be generally of high quality, there are areas of concern. Long waiting lists and times, the pressure of workload on staff, hospital closures, decaying buildings and the explicit rationing of care are all issues which have featured in the press and in general public debate. There is no doubt that some of the increased criticism has been fuelled by the reforms introduced to the NHS. The increased emphasis on competition which accompanied these reforms has been seen by some to be misplaced; others have argued that the reforms will introduce a two-tiered service into the NHS. The objective of the reforms, to increase efficiency, has misdirected the argument for some, particularly, it would appear, those working in the NHS. They argue that efficiency is defined purely in terms of throughput rather than improvements in health. Perhaps not surprisingly, against this critical background there has been a widely expressed opinion that the real issue with health care in the UK is one of underfunding.

Certainly health care expenditure, as with all UK public expenditure-based programmes, has been subject to increased scrutiny over the recent past. The general emphasis on the control of public expenditure has meant that the whole public sector has seen expenditure growth maintained within tight limits. Whether this translates into underfunding in any particular area of expenditure is, however, a different issue. The general difficulty is that the debate on funding hardly ever gets past a discussion of expenditure levels. It is rare to consider what that expenditure buys, and even rarer to consider whether the purchase has any value. A presumption of underfunding does not amount to evidence.

It is, of course, extremely difficult to define the optimal level of health care expenditure. One of the basic problems is the difficulty of expressing the objectives of the health care sector in an explicit manner. Efficiency is often stated as an objective, but is seldom defined. Equity is also still seen to be a major consideration in the resource allocation process, but again it is hardly ever explicitly defined (see Le Grand's chapter in this volume). Yet until the objectives are clearly outlined, it is impossible to state whether health care is under- or overfunded. Many of the arguments that are frequently offered in support of underfunding are misleading, generally supporting long-held biases in perspective or confusing the issues involved. This chapter addresses the question of underfunding, through considering what is commonly meant by underfunding and how the optimal funding of health care can be attained.

Some history

Underfunding in the health care sector was not an issue until at least the 1960s. Discussion on health care expenditure during the 1950s was concerned with containing, rather than increasing, health care expenditure. This concern was shown to be misplaced; the Guillebaud Committee reported on the common presumption that expenditure on the NHS was rising too fast and threatening to dominate public expenditure (HMSO 1956). This report drew attention to the fact that, after taking account of price inflation in the health care sector, real rates of expenditure were growing at a slower pace than commonly believed and dampened the concern.

Since 1960 the nation has been devoting increasing amounts of national resources to health care. Table 7.1 shows expenditure on health care as a percentage of GDP for various years. As can be seen, over the 30-year period there has been a slight but steady increase in the UK's national resources which have been given over to health care. This increase indicates that the income elasticity, defined as the proportionate change in expenditure given a proportionate change in national income, is greater than 1 – a 1 per cent increase in GDP is associated with a greater than 1 per cent increase in health care spending.

Table 7.1   Total UK health care expenditure as a percentage of GDP

Year	1960	1965	1970	1975	1980	1985	1990
Expenditure	3.9%	4.1%	4.5%	5.5%	5.6%	5.8%	6.1%

Source: OECD (1993).

This is confirmed by Table 7.2 which shows that real expenditure growth in the UK has generally been higher than overall GDP growth. Indeed, as can be seen, in no period was real health expenditure growth lower than the growth rate of GDP. The average annual growth rate of health care expenditure in the UK for the period 1970–90 was 3.9 per cent, which contrasts with the 2.2 per cent average annual growth rate of real GDP.

These trends appear to be somewhat at odds with the belief that health care is underfunded. We are, as shown, devoting slightly more of national income to health care each year. It could be suggested that an even greater share of

Table 7.2   Health care expenditure growth, average annual growth rates

	1960–65	1965–70	1970–75	1975–80	1980–85	1985–90	1970–90
	Real health care expenditure growth						
UK	4.4	4.3	6.1	2.9	2.7	3.9	3.9
Germany	6.1	7.0	9.0	4.0	1.7	1.6	4.0
France	10.2	7.7	7.0	4.9	3.8	3.8	4.9
US	7.3	7.4	4.9	5.4	5.7	6.1	5.5
Canada	7.7	8.2	5.6	4.4	5.9	4.2	5.0
	Real GDP growth						
UK	3.2	2.5	2.0	1.8	2.0	3.1	2.2
Germany	4.8	4.1	2.2	3.3	1.1	3.0	2.4
France	5.8	5.4	3.3	3.2	1.5	2.9	2.7
USA	4.8	2.8	2.2	3.2	2.9	3.0	2.8
Canada	5.7	4.6	5.2	3.9	2.9	3.0	3.8

Source: OECD (1993).

GDP should be allocated to health care. Indeed the ratio of health care expenditure to GDP has remained relatively stable from 1975 onwards, bringing it closer to the growth rate of GDP generally. So one argument might be to increase the allocation of resources to health care to restore the higher rates of increase in expenditure which were experienced in the 1960s and early 1970s. Reliance on restoration of historical rates of growth as the sole justification for increased expenditure has little real defence.

Another, equally simple, argument states that the UK spends less than other countries and is therefore underfunding health care. From Table 7.2 it can be seen that, in comparison to other countries, the UK's rate of growth health care expenditure is indeed relatively low. Instead of being seen to be an advantage – the UK has been more successful in containing health care expenditure growth – some duly see this as evidence of underfunding. But in fact such comparisons tell us little.

The basis of this argument normally rests on regressing health care expenditure per capita on GDP per capita to compare relative expenditure across different countries. Notwithstanding the difficulties in making like-for-like comparisons, some interpretations of these data highlight that because the UK mapping of health care expenditure per head against GDP per head lies below the estimated regression line that best fits these data, this can be taken as indicative that too little is being spent on health care. Yet such an interpretation does not necessarily follow.

Regression operates on the basis of random variation. In other words, some observations will lie below and some above the regression line. The interpretation that because an observation lies below the regression line it is evidence of underspending involves a value-judgement that observations that lie on the line are somehow 'appropriate'. Other than defending some form of average expenditure, it is unclear what argument is being invoked.

Prices and quantities

Such simple arguments do not give any indication about the degree of underfunding, if any, experienced by the health care sector. Some illumination may be gained through recognition that expenditure is merely price multiplied by quantity. Underfunding could then arise either because prices are not rising quickly enough or because, given prices, not enough health care is being produced, i.e. quantity is not growing fast enough. Such a decomposition helped the Guillebaud Committee dispel doubts of overfunding in the 1950s (HMSO 1956). It may equally aid the analysis of underfunding.

This decomposition of expenditure is, of course, a statistical identity applied to expenditure data and tells us little about the underlying behavioural trends. Indeed the quantity series is defined by dividing the expenditure series by the relative price series thereby imbedding any measurement error. Table 7.3 breaks down real health care expenditure in the UK for the past three decades into relative price and quantity movements. The relative price figures reveal whether prices in the health care sector are growing at a faster rate than in the economy generally. The quantity figures show whether output is growing faster in this sector than in other sectors.

Table 7.3 UK health care expenditure: relative prices and quantities, average annual growth rates

	1960–65	1965–70	1970–75	1975–80	1980–85	1985–90	1970–90
Health care expenditure growth minus GDP growth	4.4	4.3	6.1	2.9	2.7	3.9	3.9
Relative prices	8.7	–9.5	–1.5	0.5	0.7	1.7	0.3
Volume	–4.0	15.3	7.7	2.4	2.0	2.1	3.5

Source: OECD (1993).

Relative prices

Taking relative prices first, this effect appears to have been fairly small over the period as a whole, particularly in the recent past. Over the period 1970–90 prices in the health care sector rose on average by 0.3 per cent more per annum than in the economy as a whole, although it is true that for the last period, 1985–90, the average differential was 1.7 per cent.

Health care expenditure growth driven solely by price growth might imply that the health care sector was experiencing higher inflation rates than the rest of the economy. There would be no real gain from the increased expenditure on health care if it was merely fuelling price increases. Increased expenditure could, if it was generating relatively high rates of health sector inflation, be consistent with a view that the sector was underfunded as there would be no real growth. This, however, does not appear to have been the case given the relatively small price differential.

Alternatively, relative price growth could be a reflection of productivity in the health care sector differing from that in other sectors. Some economists, including Fuchs (1968) and Baumol (1967), have argued that productivity growth in service sectors, such as the health care sector, is likely to be lower than in the manufacturing sectors of the economy. The basis of this argument is that technology changes which allow the substitution of capital for labour provide the main source of productivity growth, and that the scope for such changes in the service sector is limited as the service sector is labour-, rather than capital-intensive. Therefore productivity in the service sector will lag behind that in the manufacturing sector.

This slower-than-average growth in labour productivity in the service sector will mean higher than average costs, as labour costs keep pace with those in the manufacturing sector. If the demand for services is relatively price-inelastic, then as the economy expands the service sector's share of total employment will increase. Coupled with relatively high average costs, this means increasing expenditure on the service sector over time.

If this were the case then growth in health care expenditure which was higher than GDP growth could, again, be consistent with a view that the sector was underfunded. The expenditure rises would be associated with increasing relative health sector costs over time, with little real gain in output.

If applied to the health care sector this explanation would rely on differential labour productivity to explain some of the rise in health care prices over time. The health care sector is labour-intensive. The issue of relative productivity differentials is therefore concerned with the ratio of total employment to total output over time. Over the period 1970–90, employment in the UK health care sector employment grew by 2.39 per cent per annum as compared with 0.5 per cent per annum in the rest of the economy – a differential trend in the rate of growth of employment of 1.79 per cent. During this period, the health sector achieved output growth that was only 1.3 per cent higher than the economy generally.

In other words, employment growth was relatively higher in the health care sector and was also higher than the relative growth in output achieved by that sector. These crude figures suggest that productivity did lag behind the rest of the economy, but not by much. The implied lagging of productivity is enough to account for the small but positive differential trend in prices.

Differences in relative prices between the health care sector and the rest of the economy appear to have been small. Any growth in health care expenditure relative to national income is not explained by relative price movements. The relative growth in expenditure has not been dominated by higher rates of inflation or significantly lower rates of productivity within the health care sector. Consequently, the conclusion is that any increase in expenditure has been real rather than nominal and the impact of lower productivity gain has not led to excessive price increases in the sector.

Relative quantities
As indicated by Table 7.3, the largest growth in expenditure is associated with relatively high rates of volume growth. Overall growth in health care expenditure was 3.9 per cent during the period 1970–90, and was dominated by a 3.5 per cent rise in the volume of services delivered. This raises the apparent paradox of increased volume of service delivered but a view that underfunding exists. If the UK health care sector is underfunded, then it can only be because the increased volume of health care provision has been outstripped by the demands placed on the sector.

In analysing volume increases it is necessary to remind ourselves that the volume of service delivered is obtained by dividing real expenditure by relative prices. Such volume figures are clearly not a true measure of either the real input quantity or quality associated with the sector, but a mere proxy of the volume of service delivery. Bearing this proviso in mind, the high rates of growth in the volume of health care resources relative to the rest of the economy are sometimes explained by increased servicing to match the demand for health care arising from an ageing population and by implementation of more expensive technology.

NHS expenditure incorporates an amount that explicitly allows for the increased resources that are held to be a result of an ageing UK population. Estimates of the demand for hospital and community services that are directly a result of demographic pressure is based on per capita expenditure on different age groups. The Social Services Committee (1988) gave precise estimates of the expenditure associated with these population trends, which are reproduced as Table 7.4.

Table 7.4 Estimates of demographic pressure on health care expenditure

Year	Predicted increase in demand as a result of demographic pressure (%)
1988/89	1
1989/90	1
1990/91	0.9
1991/92	0.7
1992/93	0.5

Source: Social Services Committee (1988).

There is increasing evidence, however, that the demography of the population *per se* does not radically alter the demand for health care. What matters is not the ageing of the population itself, but rather the increased intensity of health care resource use as individuals grow old and, importantly, the fact that this intensity appears to have been increasing over time. Bosanquet and Gray (1989) present some evidence that this is the case in the UK. They find that in considering the percentage distribution of NHS expenditure by age group for the years 1951/52, 1980/81 and 1986/87 there has been a dramatic movement in expenditure toward the elderly. Total expenditure of NHS resources on those aged 65 and over was 20 per cent of total expenditure in 1951/52, but had risen to 49 per cent by 1986/87. Per capita expenditure on the over-75s rose from just over twice the average expenditure per person to almost five times the average. This movement in expenditure had been achieved through a falling proportion of expenditure on the 15–64 age group, where NHS expenditure was halved from 60 per cent of total expenditure in 1951/52 to less than a third in 1986/87.

Such expenditure movements cannot be explained by demographic changes alone. In 1960 the proportion of the UK population aged over 65 was 11.7 per cent. This had increased by 1990 to 15.8 per cent. For the over-75s the percentages are 4.2 in 1960 and 7 in 1990. The increase in resource use appears to generally reflect greater intensity of health care resource use for these age groups over time. This increased expenditure on the elderly appears, largely, to be a consequence of higher rates of usage in hospital resources by the elderly. As Bosanquet and Gray state, 'older people are admitted to hospital at a much higher than average rate, but also this difference has been widening over the last two decades or so' (1989, p. 14).

The important point is that demand *per se* is not driving this expenditure growth, but increased use of health care services by the elderly. This use is regulated by the suppliers of health care – it is supply-led rather than demand-led. It is difficult, then, to reconcile underfunding with increased demand being placed on the system, if the demand is defined by the suppliers. It is difficult, in any sector of the economy, to take seriously arguments from the suppliers that there is underfunding, especially in a sector where most expenditure converts into the supplier's income.

That said, let us assume that 1 per cent of the growth in the volume of health care resources can be traced to increased demands placed on the sector due to demographic effects. Given a relative growth in volume which was 3.5 per cent higher than the economy generally, this leaves 2.5 per cent unaccounted for.

It may be that there is indeed more that can be done for the elderly, and other segments of the population, as health care technology continues to improve. There is certainly a belief that such technology increases, rather than decreases, expenditure. This may be because the technology is itself inherently expensive or because technology complements, rather than substitutes for other inputs in the medical production process. Unfortunately little is known about this matter.

Weisbrod (1991), in considering US health care expenditures, has suggested that the growth in expenditure has stemmed, not from increased prices for existing technology, but rather from the high price associated with new technology. New technology has both driven up the unit cost of care and the range of services available to patients. Moreover, Weisbrod implies that health care systems which have prospectively allocated funds have been better placed to control such expenditure pressures than systems, like the US health care sector, which have historically allocated funds by retrospectively reimbursing incurred costs.

Generally the system operated by the UK health care sector is one where aggregate funds are allocated prospectively in line with Treasury estimates of growth in GDP. So total expenditure on health care in the UK, unlike the US, has always faced an aggregate budget constraint. This system does, however, impose its own costs. It may be that UK health care is not as technically advanced as that in the US as a result of this budget constraint. Some of the presumption of underfunding may come from lower technological growth than in other countries.

Indeed, in recognition of the budget restriction on technological growth, the Department of Health has historically been allocated somewhere between 0.5 per cent and 1 per cent of funding specifically for technology growth. The point remains, though, that the aggregate expenditure constraints on health care do limit the ability of new technologies to push up expenditure levels.

Returning again to consider overall health care expenditure and the relative growth of volume of health care resources, taking another 1 per cent as representing expenditure for technology growth which is specific to this sector, the sector has still witnessed a 1.5 per cent higher growth rate in the volume than other sectors of the economy during the period 1970–90.

It would appear, then, that expenditure on health care has grown, and at a faster rate than national income and, by implication, at a faster rate than other sectors of the economy on average. This growth in health care expenditure appears to have funded an increased volume of service delivery, rather than being lost in cost increases arising from relatively high prices or low productivity which were specific to the sector. Moreover, the increased volume of service growth remains even after accounting for the greater demands placed on the sector from the greater intensity of use by the elderly or from the funding of new technologies.

It is certainly the case, then, that while real expenditure has been increasing, after taking account of differential prices and, more importantly, the demands placed on the sector, growth has been limited. While the growth in volume of service delivered, adjusted for the impact of demography and health technology, has not been substantial, it does nevertheless seem somewhat at odds with the view that the sector is underfunded.

Expenditure versus opportunity cost

Of course expenditure patterns themselves hardly ever reveal the true costs of resource use. Expenditure is a reflection of the explicit financial costs of the services rendered by health care providers, normally taken as the costs of capital and labour employed. But there are also implicit costs. In using resources within the health care sector, the production of other goods and services are forgone. The true cost of producing health care will also acknowledge the value of alternative goods and services that must be forgone to produce it.

This is the notion of opportunity cost. It was highlighted by the advertising campaign used by one of the health unions in a recent general election where the choice between more health care expenditure was contrasted with increased defence expenditure – the specific issue was whether society values a kidney machine more highly than a Trident missile. It is these trade-offs between different resource patterns both within and across sectors of the economy which determine the optimal mix of resource allocation and through this help to determine whether a sector is over- or underfunded.

Pauly (1993) has attempted to establish the opportunity cost of health care provision at the aggregate level, although even here such measures are confined to health care labour only. To initiate his analysis, he points out that expenditure is merely income when defined from another perspective. Health care expenditure is equal to the income earned by those factors of production, mainly labour, providing health care.

If there is any monopoly power held by the suppliers of health care, then the prices paid for their services will not represent merely the cost of providing these services, but also the rent or surplus gained from exploiting monopoly power. Given barriers to entry in most health care professions, and the subsequent monopoly gained over service provision, it can at least be speculated that labour in this sector earns above-normal income. Expenditure will encompass some element of monopoly return and expenditure will not be a good indicator of the opportunity cost of provision. Having noted this proviso, Pauly then calculates two measures of opportunity cost.

The first assumes the opportunity cost to any country of a unit of health care labour is approximated by GDP per worker in that economy. An approximation to opportunity cost is then the proportion of the population devoted to providing health care. To calculate this, Pauly estimates total weighted health care employment to take account of the high levels of the clinical profession's relative income. On this basis, as can be seen from Table 7.5, the UK has 5.52 per cent of its workforce engaged in producing health care services, as compared to 8.31 per cent, 7.24 per cent, 6.39 per cent and 7.03 per cent in France, Germany, Canada and the US respectively. If the opportunity cost of those workers is the same as in France and Germany, then the burden of labour costs for the UK in producing health care is lower than in these countries.

Table 7.5   Opportunity cost of health care production

	Health care employment as percent of total employment	Total expenditure on all health care labour: US wages
UK	5.52	5.09
Germany	7.24	6.56
France	8.31	6.85
Canada	6.39	4.89
US	7.03	4.77

Source: Pauly (1993).

Productivity differences between workers in these countries do exist, of course, and do affect this definition of opportunity cost. It appears conclusive, however, that manufacturing productivity, as measured by output per head, has been lower in the UK than these countries. Pratten (1990) estimates labour productivity to be 26 per cent and 38 per cent higher for France and Germany respectively in 1979. However, for the period 1980–88 the annual growth rate of labour productivity per employee in manufacturing industry was higher in the UK (4.2 per cent per annum), as compared to France (2.2 per cent) and Germany (2.9 per cent) (OECD, various years).

Moreover, the UK also had higher unemployment throughout the 1980s – 10 per cent as compared to 9.1 per cent for France and 6.1 per cent for Germany. Thus, even accepting improved productivity over the 1980s in the UK relative to other countries, it would appear that the opportunity cost of health care labour is lower in the UK than in countries such as France and Germany.

This does not tell us whether the expenditure on health care is appropriate or inappropriate. What it does say is that, under certain assumptions, the opportunity cost of producing health care is lower in the UK than in countries like France and Germany. In other words, the cost of producing health care in the UK, as measured in terms of other production forgone, is lower than in these other countries.

The second measure of the opportunity cost is based on costing health care workers uniformly across different countries – each country's health care worker is costed at US input prices. These standardized input costs are then divided by GDP (measured in US dollars) to give a ratio of the standardized cost of a health care worker to national income. This measure of opportunity cost essentially assumes that the opportunity cost of a health care worker is the same in each country and can be measured relative to the level of GDP. Again, as shown in Table 7.5, and consistent with the first measure, the UK is found to have a low opportunity cost in health care production relative to some countries.

The conclusion from Pauly's calculations is that the opportunity cost of health care labour (and by inference health care), is low in the UK. This reflects the fact that UK manufacturing productivity has been lower than that of its competitors. There is less to be given up in the UK than in other countries in the production of one unit of health care.

Returning to the Fuchs and Baumol argument outlined above, this would be consistent with the fact that service sector labour costs are relatively low in the UK. This, in turn, may give an explanation for the relatively low expenditure on health care in the UK. Health care expenditure is low because UK manufacturing productivity is relatively low and this has held down labour costs in the manufacturing sector and in other sectors of the economy.

While the opportunity cost calculations do not determine the optimal level of health care expenditure, they do highlight some important issues. For example, Pauly's calculations emphasize that, in a labour-dominated sector, expenditure converts into income. What is spent by one person becomes someone else's income. Bearing in mind that approximately 70 per cent of expenditure on health converts into labour costs, it should be noted that average health employees' earnings as a proportion of average salaries in the UK have been remarkably constant in remaining at unity over the period 1960–90. In other words average health care earnings have equalled average earnings generally throughout this period.

Yet this general picture varies depending on the specific periods and the particular class of labour considered. For example, private sector income has increased by 17 per cent more than average NHS income since 1981/82. Clinicians as a distinct employment group, however, have fared better generally with earnings remaining approximately 2.5 times higher than average earnings over this period. They constitute only 6.5 per cent of total health care employment, however. Moreover, if clinicians are compared to other professionals, their earnings do not appear to be exceptional. Wilson (1993), for example, compared rates of return for the medical profession against other professions and found that the returns gained were not very different from those of other professions. In other words, labour costs in the health care sector are not out of line with labour costs elsewhere in the economy.

What can we say generally about health care expenditure so far? Prices, which are dominated by the cost of labour in this sector, have not increased significantly over the past 40 years. This is probably because UK productivity has been relatively low and this has held down labour costs generally. At the same time health care expenditure has been rising faster than GDP generally. An increased growth in the volume of services delivered would appear to account for this. This increased growth in volume of output cannot all be accounted for by increasing demands, arising from demographic and technological changes, being placed on the system.

It would appear that we get what we can afford; possibly slightly more. As our general productivity levels are low, we have low unit costs in the health care sector. Moreover, the volume of service provision appears to have kept pace generally with the demands placed on the system – arguably growing at a slightly faster rate. In aggregate terms, expenditure has certainly outstripped income. If the system is viewed as being underfunded, there must be other reasons.

Other factors
If, as a society, we wish to spend a greater amount of our resources on health care, there is nothing wrong in doing so. It merely means that the opportunity cost of health care resources will rise, although at what rate is undetermined. But that is no reason for not increasing funding – different countries spend resources in different ways reflecting the difference in the tastes and preferences of their societies. It is these differences in tastes and preferences which dictate the differences in cultures, after all. In other words, based on tastes and preferences, it may be that spending on health should be increased. A

general view that the UK is underspending on health care may reflect a preference to spend more or to spend more on specific groups within our population.

Of course preferences may be constrained by the determination of the boundaries of the NHS, although if individuals want to purchase more health care, they can always do so if they have access to a private sector that supplements the public sector. The demand for private health care has risen substantially over time in the UK: only 1.9 per cent of the UK population held private health care insurance in 1960, 3.8 per cent by 1970, 6.4 per cent by 1980 and 11.6 per cent by 1990. Consequently expenditure on private health care insurance has risen from £4.5 million in 1960 to approximately £1.5 billion in 1990.

One argument for this increased private demand is that it is associated with an increased demand for better amenities – choice of consultant, nicer rooms, etc. Others have argued that it is the avoidance of queues which has given rise to this demand, with increased waiting lists indicating increased rationing of care, i.e. lengthening lists being caused by underfunding of public health care. The difficulty with this argument is that the link between public funding, queues, and private care is complex. Few studies have considered the relationship between public and private health care. MacAvinchey and Yannopoulos (1994) present evidence to show that private insurance is in fact a substitute for the NHS. The cross-elasticity of demand with respect to the price of private care is shown to be positive and growing, indicating a greater degree of substitutability over time. Private health care insurance does not, from this evidence, complement public expenditure on health care, but displaces it.

Additionally, it may be that society has optimistic expectations about the capability of health care to deliver output. The assumption that we are pursing optimal funding of health care encompasses the presumption that we would not knowingly use our resources in a wasteful way. Certainly some health care may do little good for the patient – tonsillectomy, haemorrhoidectomy and hysterectomy have all been shown to be of little benefit for specific groups of patients (Roos 1979; *The Lancet*, 1975; Sandberg et al. 1985). Identifying the value that is obtained from specific interventions remains a complex task. The additional benefit arising from additional expenditure on individual therapies is an underdeveloped area of evaluation. Defining benefit, despite all the noise generated by such outcome measures as QALYs (quality adjusted life years gained), remains in an early stage of development. Attaching value to that additional benefit is even less developed.

An ideal system of funding would consider the additional benefit to be gained from additional expenditure. The marginal benefit of expenditure across different interventions would be constant, no matter the health outcome. Assuming marginal benefit is decreasing in expenditure, if this were not the case then welfare could be increased by transferring resources from states where the marginal benefit was at present high to states where it is low. Unfortunately it is currently not known what the precise relationship is between expenditure and benefit across most medical interventions, not least because of the difficulty in defining benefit.

In most cases we simply do not know whether further expenditure represents good value for money. We cannot, therefore, rely on information on allocations to individual interventions to dictate the optimal level of funding. Possibly as more information becomes available this may be an option. The experiments in calculating costs per QALY, or indeed costs per any unit of measure of outcome, within the health care sector can only help in this respect. For the moment, however, we remain faced with less focused choices and ultimately a decision over the aggregate level of resourcing to devote to health care.

Conclusions

The optimal level of health funding is a normative question dictated partly by the aggregate tastes and preferences of society. However, even accepting this general statement, some information can be gained about the general trend in expenditure levels. It can be shown, for example, that expenditure on health care in the UK has increased over time, arguably keeping slightly ahead of the demands placed on the sector. But given that the question is a normative one, it is not possible to state whether such growth has represented a movement towards 'acceptable' funding of health care or not.

Certainly, in as much as a number of proposals have been put forward to increase funding, it is possible that there is an acceptance that underfunding does exist, as defined as a position where society would value resources devoted to health care higher than the use of these resources in some competing manner. A basic premise of most of these proposals is that within the existing system of funding through general taxation it is unlikely that health care expenditure will rise considerably. Two basic alternatives have been suggested.

Extending charges for services is the first. This seems at odds with increasing the volume of service delivery, as in most sectors if the charge is raised, the quantity consumed falls. Indeed, this is what has happened with chargeable prescription items within the NHS. The charge for non-exempt prescriptions has risen in real terms by 260 per cent since reintroduction in 1968 with a subsequent fall in utilization from 118 million prescriptions presented to 54 million. Ignoring the obvious equity issues raised over which individuals should bear charges, or indeed whether it is justifiable to tax the sick directly, there appears to be little justification for increasing charges if this is going to reduce service utilization generally.

A second popular policy response is to introduce some form of earmarked or hypothecated taxation. This would make the relationship between the funding of health care and the expenditure levels more explicit. If it was perceived that there was underfunding, society might then be prepared to bear additional taxation to increase expenditure. A major difficulty with earmarking taxation for health care is that the commodity is valued largely for its private gain. This may distort the preference revelation, the vote, for hypothecation. Individuals would support increased funding if there was gain to them. There may, of course, be some external effects (individuals may care about others' health states or may even support the provision of health care *per se*), but whether these effects would sufficiently outweigh private interest is a disputable point. The view that if individuals know their tax is going to support the NHS, they will willingly pay higher rates, is based not so much on economics as on faith.

As this chapter has shown, simple exposition of the patterns of real expenditure is illuminating. Within the existing system of funding we are devoting increasing amounts of our national income to health care. We have, as a nation, managed to contain the rate of growth of expenditure on health care more than others. Whether this is a good or a bad indicator of performance is unclear. A number of issues remain to be resolved. Expenditure funds health care which impacts on health. However, we know relatively little about the relationship between health care and health. From a different perspective expenditure finances the incomes of the providers of health care. Again, we know little about the operation of the health care labour market. The incentives and disincentives arising from different payment schemes will have some impact on the supply of labour, but little is known about precise impacts of different schemes. It is possible to advance knowledge in these areas without addressing the fundamental issue of the value that individuals, and society generally, place on health care. Ultimately, however, the level of funding will be determined by the choices over the kind of society we wish to live in.

References

Baumol, W. (1967), 'Microeconomics of unbalanced growth', *American Economic Review*, **53**, 941–73.

Bosanquet, N. and Gray, A. (1989), *Will You Still Love Me?: New opportunities for health services for elderly people in the 1990s and beyond*, NAHA Research Paper no. 2, Birmingham: NAHA.

Fuchs, V. (1968), *The Service Economy*, New York: Columbia University Press.

HMSO (1956), *Report of the Committee of Enquiry into the Cost of the National Health Service*, Cmnd 9663 (The Guillebaud Report), London: HMSO.

Lancet (1975), editorial, 'To tie; to stab; to stretch; perchance to freeze', *Lancet*, **ii**, 645–6.

MacAvinchey, I. and Yannopoulos, Y. (1994), 'A cost approach to the choice between public and private acute health care provision', *Scottish Journal of Political Economy*, **41**, 194–211.

Pauly, M. (1993), 'US health care costs: the untold true story', *Health Affairs*, **12**(3), 152–9.

Pratten, C. (1990), *Macroeconomics*, Cambridge: Cambridge University Press.

OECD (various years), *Economic Reports*, Paris: OECD.

OECD (1993), *OECD Health Systems: Facts and Trends 1960–1991* (vols I and II), Paris: OECD.

Roos, L. (1979), 'Alternative designs to study outcomes: the tonsillectomy case', *Medical Care*, **17**,1069–87.

Sandberg, S., Barnes, B., Weinstein, M. and Braun, P. (1985), 'Elective hysterectomy: benefits, costs and risks', *Medical Care*, **23**, 1067–85.

Social Services Committee (1988), *Public Expenditure on the Social Services: a memorandum received by the Department of Health*, House of Commons Session Paper, 1987–88, London: HMSO.

Weisbrod, B. (1991), 'The health care quadrilemma: an essay on technological change, insurance, quality of care and cost containment', *Journal of Health Economics*, **24**, 523–52.

Wilson, R. (1993), 'Rates of return to the medical profession', *Journal of Health Economics*, **12**, 23–37.

8 Equity, efficiency and rationing of health care*

Julian Le Grand

Introduction

There is now a general awareness that the rationing of health care is unavoidable. With the advance of medical technology, rising incomes and a general growth in health awareness, the demand for health care is growing faster than the resources that can be allocated to it. And if more people want more care than can be met from available resources, then a process has to take place that decides who should get what. That is the rationing process, and it is one that, in the circumstances described, is inevitable.

Of course, the necessity for rationing as such is not unique to health care. Demand is likely to be greater than supply for virtually all the goods and services produced in modern economies and there has to be some kind of system for rationing them. However, health care is different from most other goods and services in that the mechanism usually used for rationing the latter has been ruled out: the price system. Most goods and services are sold to their users at a price. For those items, if demand rises faster than supply, then other things being equal, the price rises. This results in a reduction in demand by those for whom the price is now greater than the value to them of the commodity concerned, relative to what else they could do with their money. Only those whose willingness to pay for the commodity is at least as great as the price will use it. In effect, the available supply of the commodity is being rationed between people on the basis of their willingness to pay for it.

There are some kinds of health care that are rationed in this way in the UK. For instance, tatoo removals and some forms of assisted conception are not provided under the NHS in some areas (House of Commons 1995, p. xxx). More controversially, some forms of long-term care are no longer being underwritten by the NHS, with erstwhile NHS patients being required to move into means-tested local authority care. However, a social decision has been made that willingness to pay is not an appropriate principle for rationing the vast majority of health care in the UK; hence the price system as a mechanism for rationing that care has been rejected, and that care is provided

*This paper forms part of a King's Fund Institute programme of work on rationing, undertaken by my Institute colleague Bill New and myself. The paper has benefited greatly from comments by Bill New and Tony Culyer, for both of whose insights I am very grateful.

free (or largely so) at the point of use. For these zero-priced forms of care, demand exceeds supply and principles for rationing other than willingness to pay are needed.

Despite a growing awareness throughout the Health Service that (non-price) rationing is inevitable, until recently there was little sustained analysis of the possible principles that might underlie it. A number of publications in the last two years in a variety of countries have begun to fill this gap (*British Medical Journal* 1993; [New Zealand] National Advisory Committee 1994; Frankel and West 1993; [Netherlands] Government Committee on Choices in Health Care 1992; Harrison and Hunter 1994; [Swedish] Health Care and Medical Priorities Commission 1993; [UK] House of Commons Health Committee 1995). However, the overall result can seem a rather confusing picture; and this paper is an attempt to organize some of the relevant arguments into what is hoped is a somewhat more coherent one.

The basic thrust of the paper is to take some of the more well-known rationing principles and assess their merits using three basic criteria: equity, efficiency and practicality. The next section of the paper discusses these criteria in a little more detail. The following section considers possible principles for rationing, including those concerned with need, aggregate health gain, non-health-related factors, desert and entitlement, and examines their performance against the criteria. It is argued that none successfully meet all the criteria and hence that any choice of principle will depend on the relative weights given to the criteria themselves. There is a brief concluding section.

Assessment criteria

Any attempt at assessment must have some criteria for judgement. Two such criteria that immediately strike an economist as suitable are efficiency and equity; a third that perhaps ought to strike economists more often, and would certainly figure in many other analysts' lists, is practicality. A few words on each follows.

Efficiency

Although often regarded as an uncontested term, efficiency may be interpreted in a variety of different ways. Here I shall follow economists' normal usage and define it in terms of what is commonly referred to as Pareto-optimality. Under this definition, an efficient allocation of health care is one where it is impossible to re-allocate health care (or the resources devoted to it) in such a way as to make one person better off without making another worse off. In the context of health care 'better off' may be narrowly interpreted in terms of improvement in health; alternatively it may be more broadly considered in terms of improvements in individuals' overall levels of welfare, of which better health is just one contributory factor – albeit, of course, a very important one.

Pareto-type definitions of both the narrow and broad kind are not uncontested definitions of efficiency, for they incorporate values that are less innocuous than might be at first apparent (Le Grand 1991, Chap. 3). However they will suffice for the purposes of this paper.

Equity

Equity is, of course, an even more contested term than efficiency.[1] Here I do not wish to adjudicate between competing interpretations. Instead, I propose to rely on a more general procedure and to argue that, for a rationing principle to be assessed as equitable, it should not yield outcomes that offend against moral intuitions concerning what is equitable, fair or just.[2] I have explained elsewhere why, on methodological grounds, this apparently unscientific procedure for evaluating principles cannot be avoided.[3] It also has a more pragmatic rationale: any principle which leads to outcomes that those affected regard as seriously unjust or inequitable is unlikely to be sustainable as an aid for decision-making for long.

Practicality

Some authors have argued that on practical grounds the whole process of trying to find rationing principles is futile. So, for instance, Klein has asserted that 'it is positively undesirable (as well as foolish) to search for some set of principles or techniques that will make our decisions for us: the idea of a machine grinding out priorities is absurd' (1993, p. 310). More generally, Mechanic (1995), has argued against the use of explicit criteria for rationing purposes on the grounds that it is based on an 'illusion that optimization is possible'.

It is not necessary to accept Mechanic's and Klein's arguments in full to acknowledge that an important criterion for the acceptability of any rationing principle is that it must be practical to implement. So, for example, it should be relatively easy to understand, quick to apply and, perhaps most important of all, its application to a given situation should not have information requirements that are beyond the capacity of the relevant actors to fulfil.

Rationing principles

The number of possible principles that could be – and have been – used to ration health care are legion. In what follows they are grouped under the headings of need, non-health-related factors, desert and entitlement.

Need

The National Health Service was set up at least in part so that the principal determinant of the care received by patients should be their need for such care, and only that need. This suggests an obvious starting place, for the search for rationing principles should be with the concept of need, however this is defined.

But how should it be defined? Need is a slippery concept, one that many people have put much effort in trying to capture.[4] Of the many possible interpretations suggested, two stand out. The first relates the need for care to the health status of the patients concerned; the second, to their capacity to benefit from that care.

On the first interpretation, those in greatest need of health care are those who are most ill, or, put another way, those with the largest health 'deficit'. A principle of rationing based on this conception of need would give more health care to those with the larger health deficit. A more specific formulation of this principle might be:

P.1   Health care should be allocated between patients according to the size of their health deficit.

One version of this principle is the 'rescue principle' (as formulated, and attacked, by Dworkin 1994) whereby everything should be sacrificed to preserve life. The rescue principle is often invoked when an identified individual is in danger of dying: a child in need of a liver transplant, or a potholer stuck in a cave with a broken leg. Such single cases can absorb very large amounts of resources, but nonetheless apparently acquire top priority if well publicized.

Obvious practical problems arise in defining the idea of 'health deficit'. Does it refer to pain or distress? To 'closeness to death'? What about length of time spent waiting for treatment? Also, there is the practical question as to who determines the degree of health deficit: the doctor, the hospital manager – or the patient him/herself?

Even if the practical problems could be overcome, consistent application of this principle would lead to unacceptable outcomes by reference to our other criteria. For instance, as with its application in the form of the rescue principle, it would imply that someone who is terminally ill (presumably the ultimate health deficit) should receive maximum health care, regardless of the likely outcome of that care. This could result in massive quantities of care being devoted to patients with no realistic chance of recovery; an allocation that would certainly be inefficient, and perhaps also inequitable with respect to those who were less ill – in the sense of not being terminally ill – but who could have benefited from the resources concerned had they been employed in a different way.

In fact, it has been argued both that this principle of rationing is one already employed in many medical systems and that it is indeed seriously wasteful. A recent report concluded that too many operations were being undertaken in the NHS to too little effect on those close to death (National

Confidential Enquiry into Perioperative Deaths 1993). In the US it has been estimated that the mean Medicare payment for the last year of life was seven times that of all Medicare patients, and payments during the last *month* of life constituted 40 per cent of payments during the last year of life (Lubitz and Riley 1993).

More generally, a serious weakness of this principle for allocating health care from an efficiency point of view is that it concentrates solely upon the health of the potential recipient of care and not on the ability of the recipient to benefit from that care. This suggests that it might be more appropriate to interpret the need for care in terms of the likely effectiveness or efficacy of that care or, put another way, in terms of the individual patient's capacity to benefit from care. Under this interpretation, patients in greatest need are those who have the greatest capacity to benefit. This yields a second possible rationing principle:

P.2   Health care should be allocated between patients according to their capacity to benefit from that care.

P.2 leaves 'capacity to benefit' undefined. A more specific version relates capacity to benefit directly to 'health gain': that is, with the reduction in the patient's health deficit that should follow from his/her receipt of care. As we shall see later, health gain is not necessarily identical to capacity to benefit, although the two are often used synonymously (see, for example, Harrison and Hunter 1994, p. 41). Incorporating health gain explicitly into P.2 yields:

P.2a   Health care should be allocated between patients according to their potential for health gain from that care.

Practical problems that arise with this principle concern, first, the measurement of health gain itself and, second, the attribution of health gain, however measured, to any particular form of treatment. The problems with the measurement of health gain are well known and do not need repetition here. But the problem of attribution is also significant. Some writers have argued that the effectiveness of as little as 15 per cent of medical treatments have been demonstrated (Smith 1991), implying that 85 per cent either are of proven ineffectiveness or are unproven. Even where there is a reasonable degree of consensus that a treatment is in general effective, there may be uncertainty over its potential effectiveness in the case of a specific patient.

Moreover, in addition to measurement and attribution difficulties, there is a more fundamental problem with health gain on its own as a principle for rationing – or indeed more generally with capacity to benefit as a principle on its own. The difficulty can be illustrated with an example. Imagine three individuals, one of whom would benefit very slightly more from care than the other two – her illness is treatable but slightly more serious – but whose treatment would cost twice as much (and take twice as long) as that of the others. Now suppose there is only one hospital bed available: to whom should it be allocated? The health gain principle on its own would favour the 'expensive' patient, since her gain would be (slightly) greater. However, it might be considered more sensible to allocate it sequentially to the 'cheaper' patients, on the grounds that by so doing this would lead to the extraction of a much greater health gain in total from the same resources. The outcome would be arguably both more efficient (in the sense that limited resources were being used to greater effect) and more equitable, in that two people were receiving treatment rather than one. Hence allocating purely in terms of health gain in this case would be both inefficient and inequitable.

Aggregate health gain

The example at the end of the last section suggests that the set of principles for rationing health care between different patients should take account of the total or *aggregate* health gain from the limited resources available for health care. More specifically, it suggests a third principle:

P.3   Health care should be allocated between patients in such a way so as to maximize the aggregate health gain from a given set of resources.

This could be operationalized by using as the basis for rationing, the *health gain per pound*, or its inverse, *the cost per unit of health gain*. The latter is the form of rationing embodied in, for instance, the use of cost-per-QALY league tables, where different forms of treatment are ranked according to their cost per unit of health gain as measured by quality-adjusted life-years or QALYs).[5] If health care is rationed according to the cost per unit of health gain, such that treatments with lower costs per unit are given priority over those with higher costs, then more health gain in total will be achieved from a given set of resources.

Although P.3 does not suffer from the problems involving the neglect of resource constraints as P.2 (or indeed P.1), it has the same practical difficulties involving measurement and attribution, and an extra one of its own. As with P.2, implementation of the principle requires accurate information concerning the health gain to be achieved from different forms of treatment. But it also requires information concerning the *costs* of each form of treatment – no light requirement, even in the new model NHS.

However, it does meet the criterion of efficiency. Indeed, it is arguably the quintessential efficiency principle in the context of health care. If health gain is maximized from available resources, *ipso facto* it will be impossible to reallocate resources in such a way as to make one person better off (in terms of health gain) without making another worse off.

On the other hand, its success with respect to the efficiency criterion does not always carry over to the equity one. As so often with efficiency principles, its application under certain circumstances can produce outcomes that seem intuitively inequitable or unfair. For instance, it is often the case that the poor respond worse to medical treatment than wealthier people with the same condition – because the latter are better fed, live in more salubrious housing, and have superior support systems at home. In that situation, treatment of rich individuals might have a lower cost per QALY, or a higher health gain per pound than treatment of poor individuals in the same state of ill-health. Now, if individuals are weighted equally in the process of aggregating health gain (that is, a QALY is treated as the same, whether accruing to a poor or a rich individual), then allocating health care on the basis of health gain per pound or cost per QALY will result in giving the wealthy priority over the poor – not an outcome that everybody would regard as fair. However, it should be noted that this result does depend on the assumption that individuals are weighted the same, a point to which we shall return.

Another example of a potentially unfair outcome resulting from the application of this rationing principle with equal weighting of individuals concerns elderly people. If capacity to benefit or health gain is measured by QALYs, for instance, or indeed by any measure that involves years of life gained by treatment, this is likely to discriminate in favour of younger people. A life-saving treatment given to a baby, for example, would result in a larger number of life-years gained than if the same treatment were given for the same condition to a 60-year-old (or a 40- or a 20-year-old). More generally, other things being equal, life expectancy would dominate rationing procedures – again, not necessarily an outcome that everyone would consider fair.

Finally, for life-threatening diseases, this principle with equal individual weights could discriminate against disabled persons – again especially if QALYs or related measures of the quality of life were used to measure capacity to benefit and QALYs are weighted equally regardless of to whom they accrue. Other things being equal, the QALY measurement procedure attributes fewer QALYs to disabled people than able-bodied persons of the same overall life expectancy. Hence treating a disabled person for a life-threatening disease not related to his/her disability would generate fewer QALYs than the same treatment given to an able-bodied person with the same disease. The result would be a higher cost per QALY and therefore a lower priority for the disabled patient.[6]

Non-health-related principles

The three principles considered so far all involved rationing solely by patient health-related factors such as health deficit or health gain. However, the examples used at the end of the last section to 'test' the equity of the rationing outcome introduced into the discussion aspects of the patients concerned that were not directly to do with their health status, or at least not to do with the illness for which the rationing decision has to be made. These aspects included their socioeconomic circumstances (poor or rich), their age and their degree of disability. This raises a broader question: should non-health-related factors, of which these are examples, affect the rationing decision, and if so in what way?

The number of possible factors that could be included are many. The more prominent include age, gender, race, religion, doctor preference, sexual orientation, income, class, disability, personal and political influence, and contribution to others.

The equity criterion would almost certainly rule out some of the more disreputable of these possibilities. No-one would argue that nepotism, cronyism or other forms of personal or political influence would be fair ways of rationing. It is unlikely that such 'principles' would be efficient either – although it should be noted that, given their prevalence in many rationing situations outside the health arena, their use does not seem to raise practical difficulties! Equally, for most people, equity considerations would rule out rationing based on religious affiliation or sexual orientation.

Doctor preference is a little more difficult. One of the reasons why doctors may prefer to treat some patients over others is because the former may be more medically interesting. If translated into action, this preference would probably be inequitable, according to most intuitively acceptable interpretations of the term. However, if it led to improvements in medical knowledge and experience, or even if it only contributed to doctor morale, it could lead to an improvement in efficiency.

Race, gender, disability, and socioeconomic status raise more complicated issues. Again, few would seriously contend that these factors on their own ought to be factors in rationing decisions, at least if by so doing the outcome would be *negative* discrimination: that is, discrimination against already disadvantaged groups. That would undoubtedly be regarded as inequitable although, as has been noted above, in the case of socioeconomic status at least, it might be efficient.

However, that is not the end of the argument. Is there a case for some of these non-health factors, particularly those which can lead to political, social and economic disadvantage such as race, gender, income, social class and disability, being used as the basis for *positive* discrimination in rationing? That is, other things being equal, might equity require that health care for the poor, for ethnic minorities or for women, for instance, be given priority over health care for the better off, for the white population or for males – on the grounds that this offered them some compensation for their disadvantage?

If so, one way of incorporating these considerations would be to 'weight' the units used to measure health deficit or capacity to benefit, according to the extent of disadvantage associated with the person concerned. Thus, for instance, QALYs that accrue to individuals from disadvantaged backgrounds could be given a greater weight than QALYs that accrue to those from more privileged circumstances. More generally, this could be formalized as a version of principle P.3:

P.3a   Health care should be allocated between patients so as to maximize weighted health gain, where the weights attached to the health gain for different categories of patient reflect economic and social disadvantage.

The idea of weighting measures of health gain is controversial; Williams, for instance, has explicitly rejected it for use with that particular measure, arguing that 'a QALY is a QALY is a QALY' (Williams 1988). However, others have been more open to the idea. Recently, for example, weights were used by the World Bank (1993) in calculating disability-adjusted life-years in order to assess the overall burden of disease.

However, the weights used by the World Bank did not reflect an equity concern for disadvantage or for some of the other considerations mentioned above. Rather they were based on another non-health-related factor that it has been argued should be taken into account when considering rationing: the economic, social and family contribution of the individual concerned. So, for example, it might be argued that parents with young children receive treatment before childless people with otherwise the same need for the treatment. Similarly carers for the elderly, workers, or household bread-winners might be given priority. Even more broadly, some might consider that people who make a contribution to the community (Nobel prize winners, political leaders) ought to take priority, while those who 'cost' the community (alcoholics, beggars) ought to fall to the bottom of the list.

It is unlikely that the last of these at least would meet the equity criterion; it might fall foul of the practicality one as well (is it really possible to identify all those who make a broad contribution to the community?). However, the issue of dependents is more difficult. In theory this type of consideration could be taken account of by using one of the principles involving 'capacity to benefit' and defining 'benefit' so as to include not only the benefit to the individual concerned, but also that to his/her dependents. On this interpretation, those with dependents would, other things being equal, have a greater 'capacity to benefit' than those with none; hence application of a capacity-to-benefit principle (*P.2, P.2a, P.3, P.3a*), with these benefits included, would indeed give priority to the former over the latter. The World Bank's weighting procedure could be viewed as a crude adjustment for this.

This procedure also comes closer to acceptability on efficiency grounds, especially if 'better off' in the Pareto-optimality definition of efficiency is interpreted in the broad sense of welfare improvement. If people who have dependents are given priority for treatment over those without dependents then, other things being equal, the welfare of the community as a whole is likely to be raised.

The practicality argument also has some purchase here, especially when compared with some of the other grounds for discrimination that we have been considering. In the case of race or gender, the decision-maker has to make a case for discrimination on probabilistic grounds; for it would not always be easy to decide in specific cases whether the patient concerned was herself suffering from discrimination. In the case of dependents, however, the relevant facts for each individual case would be much easier to establish.

Finally in this section, the question of age. It was noted above that the use of most measures of capacity to benefit tend to favour the young over the old, simply because they have a longer life expectancy and hence the period over which they benefit from any particular course of treatment is likely to be longer. Should we use rationing principles that are more even-handed with respect to age?

It should be noted that this age 'bias' implicit in capacity-to-benefit principles is simply a consequence of trying to calculate capacity to benefit appropriately; the years of benefit for younger people of a life-saving course of treatment are simply greater in number than those for older ones. Moreover, even if the principle does have an unintended bias in favour of the young, there might be an argument that such a bias is justifiable, at least from an equity point of view. By definition, elderly people have had a 'good innings' at least in terms of longevity; it could be argued that it is not unreasonable to give priority in treatment to those in the middle of their innings, so to speak, or, even more, to those whose innings has only just begun. Indeed this may be a view shared by elderly people themselves (Williams 1988). On the other hand, the fact that elderly people only have a relatively small part of their innings left could be an argument for making the rest of their lives of as high a quality as possible.[7]

Desert

A rather different kind of principle for rationing health care is to allocate treatment according to desert: that is, as to whether patients are 'deserving' or 'undeserving'. In recent years, this issue has arisen particularly with respect to 'self-induced' diseases. If people deliberately take health risks in the full knowledge of those risks, should they not be held responsible for any adverse health consequences that ensue? Are they not in a sense less deserving than those who contract an illness because of factors entirely beyond their control, and hence should they not be given a lower priority for treatment? Cases that raise these kinds of issue and that have recently attracted a great deal of attention concern the treatment of smokers for conditions that have been brought on by smoking; other examples include skiing or other dangerous sporting injuries; self-inflicted injuries due to drunken driving, and so on.

At first sight the case for rationing in this way seems quite seductive. The present author has pointed out that the ways in which the terms fairness or equity are conventionally used often embody concerns about the choices open to the individuals involved (Le Grand 1991). A situation where one individual is in a worse state than another because of factors entirely beyond his/her control is commonly regarded as unfair or inequitable; however, if the difference in individual states is the consequence of freely made choices, then the situation is likely to be regarded as fair.

However, even if this argument is accepted, it does not necessarily imply that these considerations should inform the rationing decision. This is for two reasons. First, there is the sheer impracticality of asking those undertaking the rationing process to ascertain in each case of ill-health the extent to which the ill-health was brought on by factors beyond individual control. Second, it could be argued that the principle itself does not imply that people should bear the *full* consequences of the voluntary assumption of health risks. Rather it requires that they bear the 'expected value' of those consequences; and, as has been argued elsewhere (Le Grand 1991, Chap. 7) the appropriate way to do this is through the *finance* of the system, not the delivery of it.

Entitlement

Finally, there is a view that the NHS can be seen as a kind of social contract between the citizens of the UK, a contract that gives everyone the same entitlement to treatment. On this view, there should be no systematic discrimination on any grounds on the allocation of health care. If there is not enough to go round then some random method of allocation should be undertaken, such as first-come, first-serve, or, if that is regarded as not sufficiently random, by some other, truly random, procedure (Harris 1988). More formally:

P.4   Health care should be allocated between people of equal need on a
random basis.

A version of this could relate entitlement to the payment of taxes. Those who have paid taxes might argue that they are entitled to receive treatment under the NHS, since the NHS is partly paid for out of those taxes. However this would carry with it the implication that those who have not paid taxes should not receive care, which might not be so readily acceptable.

P.4 could be advocated both on the grounds of equity (in the sense that lotteries or random selection might be regarded as fair) and on the grounds of practicality (in that it avoids the information requirements of most of the other principles). However it is unlikely to be efficient, since it makes no concession to capacity to benefit, and hence its application could be very wasteful in terms of resources.

Moreover, the practicality argument is suspect. Any allegedly random procedure is open to distortion. To ensure genuine randomness, it would be necessary to have elaborate enforcement procedures to make sure that the allocations were truly random and not the result of, e.g., whim or prejudice. Hence some of the practical advantages would be lost.

Conclusion

What is apparent from the discussion is that there is no principle that will simultaneously meet all three of the criteria of efficiency, equity and practicality. To choose one principle therefore means making a trade-off of one of these criteria for the others. So choosing *P.3* (maximizing aggregate health gain) means a sacrifice of equity on the altar of efficiency; *P.4* (random allocations) means sacrificing efficiency on the grounds of a possibly dubious practicality. The choice of rationing principle will therefore depend on the relative weights the person or persons making the choice place on these criteria; and the choice that is eventually made will reveal the values of the chooser.

One final point. The paper opened with the now familiar assertion that the rationing of health care is unavoidable. This is premised in part on the assumption that the demand for health care is growing inexorably, and will continue to do so for the foreseeable future. Now, while it is undoubtedly true that rapidly growing demand is a conspicuous feature of the contemporary landscape and while it is also true that there is little that can be done to change this situation in the short term, it is perhaps not necessary to be so fatalistic about the longer term. There is currently a great deal of interest in health promotion; if the relevant measures work as they should, the overall incidence of certain diseases may be reduced and with it the demand for curative medicine for those diseases. The growth in demand is also fuelled in part by exaggerated expectations of what medicine can do; the increased attention now being paid to ascertaining the actual effectiveness of different treatments may lower those expectations and thereby in the long run reduce demand. The need to ration health care may not be with us for ever.

Notes

1. For a detailed discussion of some of the more specific interpretations in the health care context and their implications for resource allocation, see Culyer and Wagstaff (1993). My own views on the appropriate way to define equity in the general context of the economic problem are spelt out in Le Grand (1991).
2. For the purposes of this paper, the terms equity, fairness and justice are used synonymously.
3. Le Grand (1991, Chap. 4).
4. See, for example, Williams (1978), Culyer (1995), Culyer and Wagstaff (1993), and Doyal and Gough (1991).
5. See, e.g., Williams (1985).
6. This does not apply in the case of non life-threatening diseases. For in these cases, if other things are equal, then the capacity to gain QALYs is the same for disabled and able-bodied people, even if their eventual health status is different.
7. So, for instance, a surgeon told me that he once gave a high priority to a cataract operation for an elderly woman with only a year to live, so that she could enjoy that last year to the full.

References

Bell, J.M. and Mendus, S. (1988), *Philosophy and Medical Welfare*, Cambridge: Cambridge University Press.
British Medical Journal (1993), *Rationing in Action*, London: BMJ Publishing Group.
Culyer, A.J. (1995), 'Need: the idea won't do – but we still need it', *Social Science and Medicine*, **40**(6), 727–30.
Culyer, A.J. and Wagstaff, A. (1993), 'Equity and equality in health and health care', *Journal of Health Economics*, **12**, 431–57.
Doyal, L. and Gough, I. (1991), *A Theory of Human Need*, London: Macmillan.
Dworkin, R. (1994), 'Will Clinton's plan be fair?', *New York Review of Books*, 13 January, 20–25.
Frankel, S. and West, R. (1993) (eds), *Rationing and Rationality in the National Health Service: the persistence of waiting lists*, Basingstoke: Macmillan.
Government Committee on Choices in Health Care (1993), *Choices in Health Care*, Rijswijk, the Netherlands.
Harris, J. (1988), 'More and better justice' in Bell and Mendus (1988).
Harrison, S. and Hunter, D. (1994), *Rationing Health Care*, London: Institute for Public Policy Research.
Health Care and Medical Priorities Commission (1993), *No Easy Choices – the difficult priorities of health care*, Stockholm: Ministry of Health and Social Affairs.
House of Commons, Health Committee, First Report (1995), *Priority Setting in the NHS: Purchasing*, Session 1994–95, 134–1. London: HMSO.
Klein, R. (1993), 'Dimensions of rationing: who should do what?', *British Medical Journal*, **307**, 309–11.
Le Grand, J. (1991), *Equity and Choice: an Essay in Economics and Applied Philosophy*, London: HarperCollins (now Routledge).
Lubitz, J.D. and Riley, G.F. (1993), 'Trends in Medicare payments in the last year of life', *New England Journal of Medicine*, **328**, 1092–6.
Mechanic, D. (1992), 'Professional judgement and the rationing of medical care', *University of Pennsylvania Law Review*, **140**, 1713–54.
Mechanic, D. (1995), 'Dilemmas in rationing health care services: the case for implicit rationing', *British Medical Journal*, **310**(6995), 1655–9.
National Advisory Committee on Core Health and Disability Services (1994), *Core Services 1993/4, First Report*, New Zealand: Government Printing Office.
National Confidential Enquiry into Perioperative Deaths (1993), *Report 1991/2*, London: NCEPOD.
Rawls, J. (1972), *A Theory of Justice*, Oxford: Oxford University Press.

Smith, R. (1991), 'Where is the wisdom...? The poverty of medical evidence', *British Medical Journal*, **303**, 798–9.

Williams, A. (1978), '"Need" – an economic exegesis' reprinted in Culyer, A.J. (ed.), *The Economics of Health*, vol .1, Aldershot: Edward Elgar, 1991.

Williams, A. (1985), 'Economics of coronary artery by-pass grafting', *British Medical Journal*, **291**, 326–9.

Williams, A. (1988), 'Ethics and efficiency in the provision of health care' in Bell and Mendus (1988).

World Bank (1993), *World Development Report, 1993: Investing in Health*, Oxford: Oxford University Press.

Index

Aaron, H.J. 118
accident and emergency units 122
accidents, deaths from 40
acute wards 122
affiliative behaviour 50–51
age discrimination 156, 159, 162
Alzheimer's disease 60
American Cancer Society 94
American Child Health Association 7
anaesthetists 109, 110, 111, 114, 116, 121
Anderson, T.F. 90
appointment systems 99–100
Arrow, K.J. 77
Atkin, K. 111
Audit Commission 106, 107–8, 112
Australia
    health care expenditure as percentage of GDP 107
    intervention rates 9
Austria, health care expenditure as percentage of GDP 107
autopsies 10
average costs 94–6, 120, 121, 125, 126, 127, 130, 138

Bagust, A. 111
Baird, P.A. 53
Banstead 113
Banta, H.D. 109
bargaining, by health authorities 69–71, 85
    competitive tendering and 65–6, 74–5, 111
    with lack of information 71, 73–4
Barker, D.J.P. 59
Barker, K. 75
basal cortisol levels 47, 48–9, 50, 52, 58, 61
Baumol, W. 122–3, 138, 144
Beardsley, T. 57
Belgium
    consumer satisfaction 31

health care expenditure
    per capita 31
    as percentage of GDP 28–9, 107
health care system 24, 26–7, 28
perinatal mortality rate 31
waiting times 31
Bellinger, D. 53
benefits of health care 91–2, 94–7, 146–7, 154–5
    aggregate health gain 155–6, 161
    data required to estimate 96–7
    weighted health gain 158–9
Bevan, Aneurin 101–2
Binmore, K. 70
Birch, S. 94
Black Report (1980) 2, 35, 38, 41, 51
Blendon, R.J. 30
block contracts 78–9
blood pressure *see* hypertension
Bloor, K. 109
Bosanquet, N. 140
Bradshaw, J. 90–91
breast cancer screening 99–100
British Association for the Advancement of Science 1
British Medical Association 114
British Medical Journal 151
British Orthopaedic Association 116
bronchitis, chronic, deaths from 40
Buchan, J. 115
burden-of-illness approach 92
Bryan, J. 108
Bryan, S. 93

Calman Report (1993) 115
Cameron, H.M. 10
Canada
    Canada Pension Plan 61
    health care employment as percentage of total employment 143
    health care expenditure
        as percentage of GDP 107
        real growth of 136